Any Guru Will Do

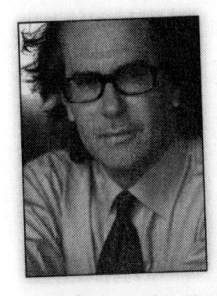

Phil Brown is a journalist who has written for a variety of newspapers and magazines including *The Sydney Morning Herald*, *The Sunday Herald Sun*, *The South China Morning Post*, *The Courier-Mail*, *The Weekend Australian* and *Griffith Review*. He is the author of two books of poetry – *Plastic Parables* and *An Accident in the Evening* – and a book of humorous travel stories, *Travels with My Angst*, which was published by UQP in 2004 and was shortlisted for the Arts Queensland Steele Rudd Award at the 2005 Queensland Premier's Literary Awards. For the past 10 years Phil has been senior writer for the lifestyle magazine *Brisbane News*. He was born in Maitland, New South Wales, but spent much of his childhood in Hong Kong, relocating to Queensland when he was 13. He lives in Wilston, Brisbane, with his wife, journalist Sandra McLean, and their son Hamish.

Other books by Phil Brown

TRAVEL WRITING
Travels with my Angst

POETRY
Plastic Parables
An Accident in the Evening

Any Guru Will Do

A modern man's search for meaning

PHIL BROWN

UQP

First published 2006 by University of Queensland Press
PO Box 6042, St Lucia, Queensland 4067 Australia

www.uqp.uq.edu.au

© Phil Brown 2006

This book is copyright. Except for private study, research,
criticism or reviews, as permitted under the Copyright Act,
no part of this book may be reproduced, stored in a retrieval system,
or transmitted in any form or by any means without prior
written permission. Enquiries should be made to the publisher.

Typeset in 12/15 pt Spectrum MT by Post Pre-press Group, Brisbane
Printed in Australia by McPherson's Printing Group

Cataloguing-in-publication data
National Library of Australia

Brown, Phil, 1956- .
Any Guru will do.

ISBN 0 7022 3542 3 (pbk.).

1. Brown, Phil, 1956- . 2. Spiritualism (Philosophy) -
Humor. 3. Life – Humor. I. Title.

128.0207

For Sandra and Hamish, always

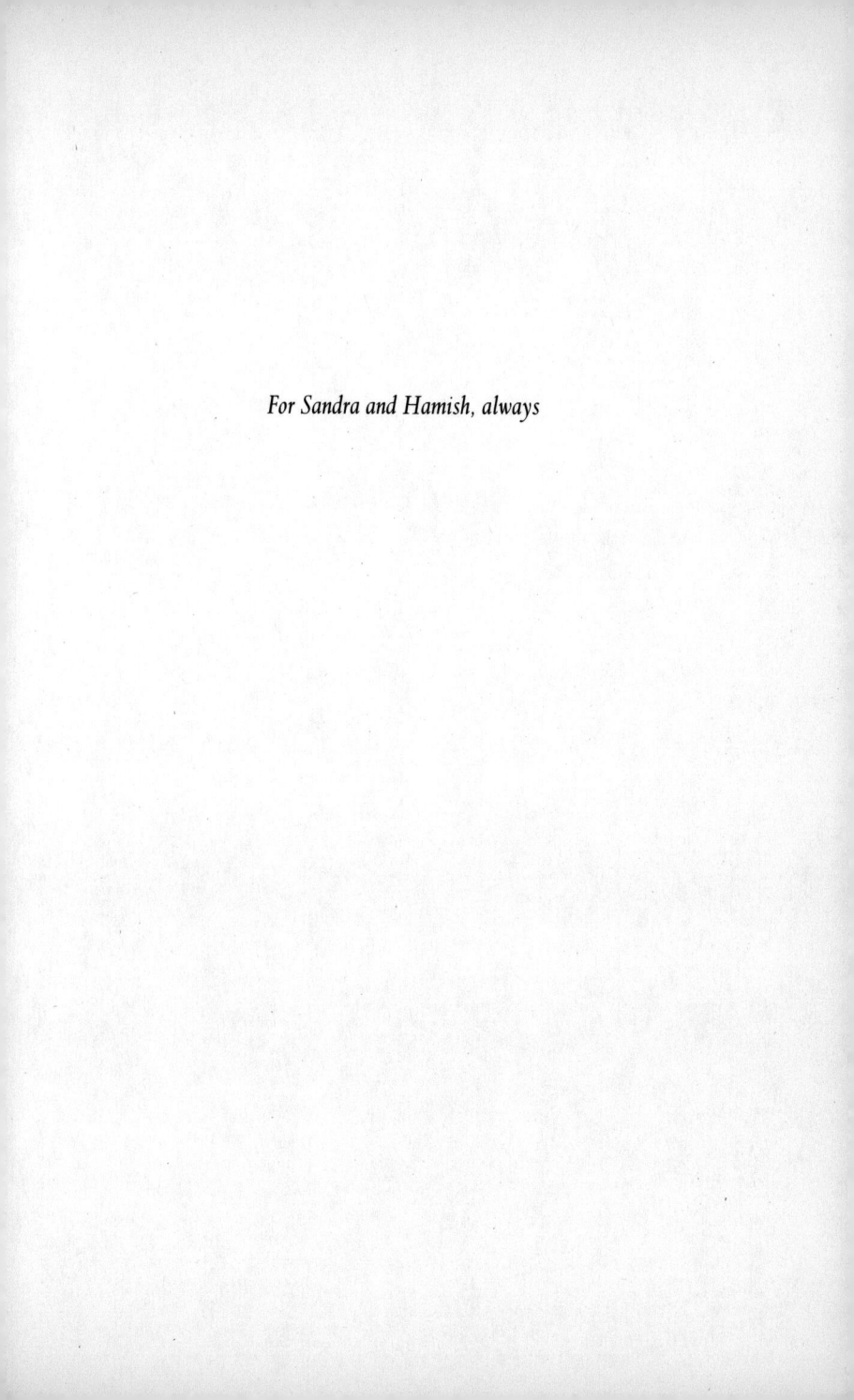

Contents

Introduction 1

In a Bard Way 4
The Pope *Will* Be Pleased 23
Clap if You Love Jesus 39
A Mantra by Any Other Name 60
On the Other Side of the Couch 81
Nil by Mouth 92
Group Grope 110
What a Bummer 121
Me of Little Faith 134
Walk like an Egyptian 145
Dr Wong, I Presume? 155
At Last, a Cure! 168
The Future, Now 183

Acknowledgements 203

Introduction

When I left high school on the Gold Coast in late 1974, graduates of my surfside alma mater were just as likely to join the Hare Krishnas or the Children of God, or become professional surf bums, as they were to go to uni or follow a serious profession. Once they had left the dusty schoolyard forever, many of my contemporaries were more interested in head-trips than in going on any real excursions into the wider world.

Woodstock and the heady days of psychedelia and Haight–Ashbury were already sort of passé by then, but Queensland took a little while to catch up. So by the time I was in my late teens, we were turning on, tuning in and dropping out – a decade late, but never mind. The Gold Coast was a sort of California-lite, where healers, quacks and mystics sprouted like mushrooms (magic, of course) after the rain, finally making their way there in the wake of the great San Franciscan awakening.

The New Age took root on the Gold Coast like nowhere

else in Australia at the time (it has since transplanted itself to Byron Bay and the surrounding hippie hills), and everything was on offer. Whether you wanted to be a Jesus freak, follow some pale imitation of the Maharishi, learn to live on thin air as a Breatharian, or turn yourself inside out with yoga, it was all on tap along the glitter strip and in the verdant hills beyond Surfers Paradise, otherwise known as Flake Central. Like many others, I drank the heady draught of this late arrival of the Age of Aquarius – or sipped it, at least. We Baby Boomers felt entitled to be able to experiment with any form of self-indulgence on offer, spiritually and materially.

Having grown up in Hong Kong surrounded by superstitious Buddhists and Taoists – where soothsayers openly plied their trade on the streets of Kowloon – I was relatively prepared for the exotica available on the Gold Coast, open to suggestion and keen to experience everything I could. At college in land-locked Toowoomba, I sought enlightenment through poetry, and sought answers to life's big questions while drinking as much beer as was humanly possible. And back on the Gold Coast, working for a cheesy-listening radio station, I flirted with evangelical Christianity, sought refuge in the bosom of the Holy Roman Catholic Church, received secret mantras, and tried everything else within reach in the search for wholeness that engulfed us all in the aftermath of the Sixties. This Boomer longing for ultimate fulfilment was encouraged by all the New Age waffle and psychobabble that we lapped up in books, courses, workshops – you name it – that pandered to the seeker and the gullible alike.

This was all an expression of my generation's existential angst, a condition I think I myself raised to an art form. It was a sort of hobby for me, and it led me a merry chase through the maze of the dawning Aussie New Age. My angst was at its most intense in the late Seventies and early Eighties, when I sought satori in some unlikely places – such as Rockhampton, more famous for its beef cattle than for spiritual illumination. But when you're a John Lennon disciple and you watch your hero seeking solace in meditation, and your primers for life are books like *The Dharma Bums* and *The Doors of Perception*, strange things can happen. And they are still happening – less frequently, maybe, but the quest goes on.

In a Bard Way

Anticipation was fast turning to despondency as we sat in the cool of the kitchen waiting to see if anyone turned up to our poetry reading. My pal in poetry, Rod, had put posters up around campus and I had carefully worded an ad for the student newspaper about our poetry evening, but so far things weren't looking good. But finally there was a rapping on the door, which echoed down the long, empty hallway.

'We're on!' said Rod as I went to the door. Two girls were standing there, a bit sheepishly, each with a folder full of what I hoped were poems.

'Hi, I'm Margie,' said the girl with long hair.

'I'm Betsy,' said the other.

'Poetry lovers, of course?' I said, partly as a statement, partly as a question. 'Come in, come in.'

I introduced Rod and we moved into the lounge room. I put Lou Reed's 'Coney Island Baby' on the turntable, ever so quietly, as background music, waited a few minutes in case anyone else turned up – no-one did – and got down to business, which was basically drinking tea and reading and talking about poetry.

'I think it's so great that people are still interested in poetry,' said Margie.

'Yes, but those people are obviously thin on the ground,' I said.

'Few are called,' said Rod with gravitas. 'And anyway, poetry is not for everyone. It takes a refined soul to appreciate poetry. Poetry is like religion, really, in its purest form. Poetry is God.'

Rod tended to make sweeping pronouncements. We all nodded. 'Anyway, are we going to read some poetry or what?' he said.

The girls each had half a dozen poems to read, and as they read we nodded knowingly. Though Margie seemed pretty chirpy, her poems were bitter and depressing. She'd obviously been studying Sylvia Plath, who was on the syllabus. Betsy's were mostly anthropomorphic nature poems in which she identified herself with natural phenomena. In one she was a tree, in another she was a rock. And the poems were full of references to wildlife, which I suspected had come from reading and, judging by the way she wrote, probably misunderstanding the work of Ted Hughes, whose poetry we were all devouring. It was all very Taoist. I tried to concentrate as they read but it wasn't easy because, basically, a poet is only ever really interested in his or her own poems, and a poetry reading is actually just a chance to strut your own stuff. Meanwhile you have to sit and look interested while your fellow poets indulge themselves.

When the girls had finished their readings, Rod read a long poem of his that I was already familiar with about woman as the underdog of history and society. It rambled a bit – or a lot, actually – and ended up with a wife tending to her violent husband, sacrificing herself completely to meet his needs. Interesting trajectory...

The girls seemed impressed. 'Wow,' said Margie.

'Wow,' said Betsy.

I followed Rod with my poems – poems that had long snaky lines because I was desperately trying to emulate D H Lawrence's poetry at the time... poems like 'Snake' and 'Bat'. One of mine, which emulated his in shape rather than subject, drew allusions between my bedroom and Calvary – my bed as the cross, dreams, my psychological crown of thorns. In another, called 'Night's Estate', I wandered a Gold Coast canal estate late at night posing questions of, I thought, some existential substance:

'What is there in this darkness men fear?
The passion they may reveal to the evening sky?
The cocktail-hour sorrows?
The loneliness of the loosened tie?'

Not exactly prize-winning stuff... but I was particularly impressed with my ending:

'Only the autumn's song of woe
Is remembered by the sky,

> And silently the white moon mouths
> It's ghostly lullaby.'

The girls seemed moved by this, but not nearly as moved as I was. A friend of mine refers to this poetic condition as being 'overwhelmed by your own sensitivity'.

After the reading we drank tea, ate biscuits and eventually broke out some cheap port. One of the girls had Gitanes, which we thought were cool and poetic because they were French. We got maudlin then as we read from books – stuff by Philip Larkin, Arthur Rimbaud, and some Bob Dylan because Dylan was 'the real poet of the street', according to Rod. We waved the girls off around ten, satisfied that the night hadn't been a total loss despite the low attendance. Rod then proceeded to crash on the couch. I went to bed woozy from the port and strong cigarettes we'd been smoking.

When I woke the following morning my mouth felt like the bottom of a budgie's cage. I went into the kitchen to make some tea, and one of my housemates, Peter, was there cooking himself eggs and bacon.

'A night on the piss always makes me hungry,' he said. 'So how did you go with those chicks last night? Did you get lucky?'

'It was a poetry reading, not an orgy,' I grunted.

'What's the use of a poetry reading if you can't get a root out of it?' he said, but I had no immediate answer to that. Besides, Rod and I spent more time thinking about poetry than girls, actually. It was a pure, virtuous, even monastic activity.

'Poetry, like virtue, is its own reward,' Rod would say.

This was late in 1976. I was 20, and had been writing poetry since high school, secretly for the most part because writing poetry wasn't exactly acceptable in the macho surf culture of Miami State High School on the Gold Coast. I was a sensitive child and an equally sensitive — far too sensitive — teenager. A huge John Lennon fan, I started writing poems influenced by his jottings. But the real outpourings came from unrequited love. I had a crush on a girl who was already spoken for, and wrote long, dire poems about this, some of which I recall giving to her, though I can't remember exactly what her response was. What I do remember is that her boyfriend arranged for his big brother to threaten me with serious physical harm if I ever went near her.

The first time I came out publicly as a poet was when I had one of my short, Zen-like pieces embedded in the bottom of my surfboard by my school friend and surfing buddy, Pete Kelleher. He got me to write my little poem on tissue paper and then he sealed it into the bottom of the board with a coat of resin. It was sort of like a haiku, something to do with the 'lonely sky' if I remember correctly. The boys down the beach were bemused and confused. Writing poetry was tantamount to declaring yourself gay to that crowd.

I certainly wasn't very literary back then, and only had a couple of books of poetry at home — one containing the verse of Rod McKuen, hardly a poet of the literary establishment. I also had a slim and depressing book of Leonard Cohen's, *The Spice-Box of Earth*. There weren't a lot of laughs in either of those volumes. My high-school English teacher had opened our eyes to the possibilities that the lyrics of the Beatles and other pop groups were, in fact, poetry. This was a revelation.

It was when I arrived at the Darling Downs Institute of Advanced Education in Toowoomba that I really started to find out more about poetry and get serious about it. I was majoring in journalism but had also chosen to do literature as an optional subject, and my tutor was Bruce Dawe. His highly accessible poems about Aussie suburbia and biting social commentaries on everything from the hanging of Ronald Ryan to the Vietnam War meant he was the best-known poet of the day in Australia – and is still widely studied. He'd even done a reading at my high school once, though I seem to recall it wasn't the happiest occasion. After reading to the unresponsive and depleted student body (there was an offshore wind blowing that day and a good swell, which signalled mass truancy), he asked if anyone had any questions, and one kid in the front row stood up and said: 'Yeah, what the hell are you doing here?' The thing that struck me about Bruce was that he didn't really look like a poet. He looked more like an army sergeant, and in fact he had once been in the air force. He was also a devout Catholic, which set him apart from a large part of the poetry pack back then, in the mid-1970s, when most bards saw themselves as the modern equivalent of the Beat generation – nihilists who thought Christianity was uncool. Buddha was acceptable but Jesus Christ? Forget about it.

The fact that Bruce was unfashionable appealed to me, because even though I wanted desperately to be a poet, I didn't want to be part of any group. It was probably dysfunctional, but I abhorred groups. I refused point blank to go on the school camps at high school because of my pathological fear of being part of a group. I fancied myself an individual – '"We are all individuals," they cried with one voice' – and recognised a model in Bruce, someone who was a bit of a maverick in his own quiet way. It was connected to that idea from the Robert Frost poem, 'The Road Not Taken', where the traveller takes the path 'less travelled by'. Frost was another poet Bruce introduced us to, which seemed very appropriate since Frost too was something of an outsider.

Rod and I were both in Bruce's class, which is how we met, kindred souls – both emotionally unstable and interested in poetry. We were inspired by Bruce's tutorials, his passion for poetry and his encyclopaedic knowledge of the subject delivered while crunching on a frequent peppermint, as he was trying to give up smoking. He didn't just know about poetry, he knew about poets, the minutiae of their lives and relationships and the social contexts in which they worked. He made poets sound like celebrities, and that helped bring the words off the page and fired our imagination and enthusiasm. With Bruce we studied Philip Larkin, T S Eliot, Sylvia Plath, Dylan Thomas, Ted Hughes, D H Lawrence ... even William Empson, who I liked because he had the coolest neck beard – make that the only neck beard – I'd ever seen. Fired up by all this, I started scribbling in earnest every night, and Rod did the same. We compared notes in the refectory before and after tutorials, and sometime during that first term decided we were going to be poets. This wasn't the sort of aspiration our parents would have been too keen on, because poetry and poverty tend to go hand-in-hand in Australia, and poets get excited when their book sales leap into double figures.

A little while after declaring ourselves aspiring poets, I asked Bruce if he would read some of my poems and give me some sort of commentary. I very nervously handed over a manila folder containing a crop of recent works. I wrote in longhand but then typed the finished product up on my rickety old Remington, puffing constantly on roll-your-own cigarettes as I pounded away. The following week Bruce brought back the poems with a covering page of notes. These contained very constructive comments about them, mostly positive and quite encouraging. This from the poetry guru! It was very exciting. Rod had done the same, with a similar result, and he was also on a high.

Even better, Bruce had asked us to come and have a cup of tea at his house on the weekend, which was like being invited to a private audience with the Pope, an appropriate allusion given Bruce's inclinations in that area.

So the following Saturday afternoon Rod and I went to Bruce's house. We were a bit nervous about the visit and felt like devotees approaching the master's ashram – in this case, a fairly ordinary house in a fairly ordinary street. When we arrived, we were somewhat surprised by the scene of suburban domesticity we discovered there. Bruce, the great bard, wasn't in his study composing verse but was, instead, up a ladder at the side of the house, wearing a pair of Stubbies and slapping on paint, while his wife, Gloria, was in the veggie garden nearby digging away, a cigarette dangling from her lower lip. Not exactly Ted Hughes and Sylvia Plath; it was more like something out of *Dad and Dave*. This was the great poet in his natural habitat? There was nothing even vaguely bohemian about the scene.

When we went inside we were offered Bushells tea and Sao biscuits smeared with Vegemite. We repaired to the lounge room so Bruce could keep an eye on the Saturday afternoon Aussie Rules football game on television — something that, as poets, Rod and I had no interest in.

In awe of the man as we were, we were surprised that such a great poet was living such an apparently ordinary life and seemed so down-to-earth. Yet his grasp of the ethereal world of poetry was so impressive and wide-ranging. His own poems could, at times, be as detached from reality as any of those by the drug-addled scribblers of the day. They soared within the context of a relatively prosaic domestic life — wife and kids — which intrigued us.

He was very encouraging, possibly because he didn't get that many prospective poets through his classes. It had been Bruce's idea that we form some sort of poetry group and hold a reading to flush any other closet poets out of the student body. He was not too surprised, though, when we told him of the outcome of our poetry evening. Poets were few and far between in Toowoomba, he reckoned.

Anyway, we were too disorganised and concerned with

our own poetry to bother about anyone else's after that first attempt. So we wrote on, showing each other poems as we went, and sometimes asking Bruce's advice, which was always generously forthcoming.

Rod, however, eventually drifted away from poetry, which I think had just been a temporary foil for his obsessive personality. Besides, he got a steady girlfriend and that really ruined things. I stuck with it, though, even after I dropped out of college and went back to the Gold Coast. I kept writing my mostly depressing poems, aping this poet and that, sending them off to various literary magazines. Bruce had encouraged me to do that, though most of what I sent out boomeranged back pretty quickly. I was rejected by the best of them ... *New Poetry*, *Meanjin* and a dozen other lofty publications. Poets often say they could wallpaper their room with their rejection slips, and I got to that point pretty quickly, which isn't really anything to boast about, I suppose. Receiving your stamped, self-addressed envelope back in the mail in under a fortnight and opening it to find a 'Dear Phil ...' rejection note is a real downer when you feel you've put your heart and soul into a poem.

I'd had a few of my verses published in student rags at college, though, which gave me some hope, and I also managed to get several poems included in a slim anthology published in Brisbane. That kept me going. Meanwhile Bruce, who I kept in touch with, had suggested I might send some to the great Les Murray, who was a friend of his: a fellow Catholic and another poet outside that bohemian fringe which always seems to colonise the poetry scene. Of course, Les is pretty famous nowadays – some might say the most famous Australian poet – and has a well-deserved international reputation. He wasn't quite as famous then but his profile was solid and building. Around this time he was co-editing one of the country's most august poetry journals – *Poetry Australia*. I bravely sent some poems off to him hoping for glory in that publication, only to have them returned a few weeks later. The difference was that instead of patronising notes about how poetry was far more than just plain narrative, Les gave constructive criticism, line by line, just as Bruce had done. And like Bruce, he was encouraging, so there was good news as well as bad news.

I went on for quite a while without an actual acceptance of a poem for publication but his words must have convinced me that success was not too far off, and due to his helpfulness I got it in my mind that I had to make a pilgrimage to Sydney to see him: to sit at the feet of the great man and soak up some poetic wisdom. I read and re-read his book *Lunch & Counter Lunch* countless times in the preceding months and was very taken with his work, which seemed to have an authenticity, like Bruce's and unlike the fashionable set.

So I had taken poetic initiation from one master and was now shaping up for an audience with another Poobah, the big fella of poetry himself. I wrote to Les of my impending trip to Sydney, asking if I might meet with him, and he very graciously told me I was welcome to visit him at his home in Chatswood on the North Shore. This was more than I had hoped for.

So I packed my poems into a tatty suitcase and booked a berth for Sydney on the old motorail service that used to run from Murwillumbah. I guess I could have flown but rail seemed more romantic, more literary, and I probably couldn't have afforded air travel anyway, since I was what a friend used to refer to as 'a poet with a liquidity problem'. I sat in cattle class, clutching my fountain pen and notebook, jotting lines for poems and occasionally dipping into the books I carried with me – a collection of Robert Graves' verse and some D H Lawrence. Plus I'd brought an anthology of Australian poetry, which included poems by Kenneth Slessor, who had written about train travel. His 'The Night Ride', one of the few poems I remember from my schooldays, brilliantly evokes a country town glimpsed from a train at night. Inspired by that, I began making notes for a future poem to be called 'Night Ride Revisited'. I had big ideas.

In the seat behind me was a young guy who, I happened to notice, was reading Joyce Cary's classic novel *The Horse's Mouth*. He was wearing paint-stained overalls and a beret, and everything about him – including his reading matter – screamed 'art student'. We got chatting. His name was Sean.

'A poet?' he said. 'Of course. You have that lean and hungry look about you. The poets I know all look like that. Are you going all the way to Sydney?'

'Yes, I'm going to visit a great poet and go to some poetry readings hopefully.'

'Sounds like a plan,' he said. 'I'm going back to art college.

My father wants me to stay in Murwillumbah and run his grocery store but that's never going to happen. I'd much rather be a starving artist.' He paused, feeling in the pocket of his overalls for something. 'Wanna scoob?'

'You can't smoke a joint in here,' I said.

'Not here, in the dunny,' he said. 'C'mon, let's celebrate in the name of art and poetry.'

There was a feeling of camaraderie in the air so I went with him, much to the disgust of an elderly gent who shook his head when he saw us both going into the toilet.

By the time we came out it was our sitting in the dining car. They used to give you tickets for staggered sittings in those days and you'd be hanging out for your turn because the seats were so damned uncomfortable, while the booths in the dining car were pretty comfy. We wobbled (in my poem 'Night Ride Revisited' I eventually evoked that wobbling by comparing it to a sailor's gait) along the passageway to the dining car. When we got there we slumped into a booth and proceeded to giggle our way through ordering a meal. We were under the influence of the herbal weed, of course, which heightened the banal experience. It was dark outside and you could sense, rather than actually see, the bush whizzing by outside. We could see our reflections in the windows, which caused more mirth.

'Have you ever looked at yourself and thought, who the hell is that?' Sean asked.

'Don't say stuff like that, I get easily freaked out,' I said, turning away. I was never very successful as a marijuana smoker. In fact, drugs in general didn't work well for me because, I have to admit, my brain was scrambled enough without them. When some of my friends started taking LSD in our last year at high school, I carefully refrained because I knew if I went on a trip I might not come back. (I know some guys who eventually didn't!) Even your common or garden variety of weed could send me into an hallucinatory state. I remember rushing out of a Mexican restaurant in Surfers Paradise once and screaming at the traffic because I was convinced the road was one way and that everyone was going in the wrong direction. 'A bad stone' was the pronouncement then and I didn't want a repeat episode now.

'No, I mean really, look at us. Who are we? What are we?' Sean asked.

'Mammals,' I said.

'Mammals with imagination, mammals with souls and mammals with a future . . . am I right?'

The conversation went on in this nonsensical way for some time, increasing in inanity, which we took for profundity in our state. The car emptied but the staff, several not-unattractive young women, let us stay on drinking tea and bullshitting into the night.

Sean and I parted at Central Station in Sydney – he to his student digs and I to my aunt and uncle's house. The first thing I did when I got there was to ring Les Murray to see if I was still welcome. He invited me to visit a couple of days later.

An audience with one of the demigods of Australian letters – this was exciting. But what would I talk about with him? Poetry, of course – but *which* poetry? I bought a second-hand copy of the *Norton Anthology of Poetry* (I already had one but that was at home) and scanned the poetry of several centuries so I could quote bits and pieces from everyone from Chaucer to Auden. I stayed up most of the night before drinking coffee and smoking cigarettes down in the back bedroom at my aunt and uncle's house. They thought I was a bit intense.

Next day, I caught a train on the North Shore line and walked from Chatswood station to his house. When I arrived there was a sense of unreality about the scene, as there had been when Rod and I visited Bruce Dawe at home. Visiting a legend has a feeling of otherworldliness about it. Again, this was a relatively ordinary suburban house in a relatively ordinary street, home to Les, his wife, Valerie, and their children. Ordinary, however, Les Murray is *not*, and I was immediately affected by his presence, his aura even, when he answered the door. It's well known that Les is a big man, large boned, of rural stock, from country New South Wales (many of his most famous poems deal with his country roots and love of the bush and rural life). Standing there in front of me, he seemed like one of those laughing Buddhas – not the serene Indian Siddhartha type but the rotund, jovial, auspicious Chinese version, the sort whose tummy you rub for good luck. I refrained from doing that.

'Come in, come in, nice to put a face to a name,' Les said jovially.

'Um, likewise,' I answered nervously.

'Come on into the lounge room,' he said. 'Would you like some coffee?'

I nodded meekly. Then the great man spread himself out along the couch, looking like some sort of Roman emperor. From a certain angle he reminded me a little of Charles Laughton, and Laughton did once play the Emperor Claudius in a film, I seemed to recall.

We drank coffee and proceeded to eat bread and cheese from a cutting board that was set in the middle of the coffee table. My God, I was breaking bread – and cheese – with one of Australia's great literary figures! He asked me about myself and my writing, and I told him about the Slessor tribute poem I'd started on the train. As I spoke about the poem I found myself leaving my body and looking at the scene, thinking, 'What a wanker you are, Phil, just shut up, will you? Les Murray is not the slightest bit interested in your pathetic doggerel.' But he nodded politely as I nervously juggled my bread and cheese, trying not to drop bits on the carpet as I did so.

'Well, that does sound interesting,' he said. 'You want to send that one along when it's finished and I'll have a look at it. I like the sound of it.'

That invitation had me floating up around the ceiling. Might the great man publish one of my poems in *Poetry Australia*? That would be the apex of all my desires, and would make up for two years of rejection and all those demeaning rejection slips. The audience continued and included a tour of the house. He showed me his writing room, which seemed extremely spartan though workmanlike. There was a rather austere-looking table, where the great bard worked, and seagrass matting on the floor.

We chatted some more but were interrupted when Valerie came home, which I took as the signal to beat a retreat. Before I went, I wanted a recommendation on some poetry readings to attend while in town. Les scratched his head for a minute and looked a bit perplexed.

'Well, I don't really go to that many,' he said. 'But you could try the Poets Union readings, which are run by Nigel Roberts. Yes, try that. Tell them I sent you.'

I seem to recall that last line being delivered with an enigmatic wink, though I wasn't sure what that indicated at the time. Les had a flyer with the details of the Poets Union's next reading and gave it to me, presumably because he wouldn't need it. I thanked him profusely and backed out the door like a slave leaving Pharaoh's throne room.

Over the next few days I spent time mooching around Sydney, browsing for hours in the antiquarian bookstores in The Rocks, where I picked up old copies of what I thought might be interesting books, like W H Davies's *Autobiography of a Supertramp*, about a hobo's travels around England. Being a poverty-stricken mendicant seemed like a romantic idea at that time.

The poetry reading Les suggested was being held upstairs somewhere in Kings Cross, so I caught a train into the city one night and trod across town to get there. The last time I'd been to the Cross, a couple of years earlier, I'd come home with a small heart tattoo on my right shoulder, none too artistically done by some guy who worked in the back of a pinball parlour. With my folder of poems I made my way there. This time I might find an audience for my work.

In a Bard Way

I had read my poems only once in public before, at college, and was nervous but hopeful. The poet Nigel Roberts was running the event. He was an established member of the Sydney literary push and a poetic-looking fellow wearing a beaten-up brown leather jacket.

'Hi, I'm Phil Brown from Queensland,' I said. 'Les Murray suggested I come along.'

'Really?' he said, turning up his nose as if I had dogshit on my shoe. 'Les is always palming people off onto us.'

The Queensland connection must have offended him. It was, after all, the height of the Joh days, and anyone who lived behind 'the banana curtain' was regarded as an apologist for that Bible-bashing bastard.

I was thrown by the cold greeting but tried to shake it off as best I could, and sat down. There was a carafe of wine in front of me so I quickly poured myself a drink and virtually sculled it, which gave me the warm glow I needed. Now I can't recall the entire line-up that evening, which is largely a blur, but as well as Nigel Roberts one name stands out – the Greek poet from Melbourne, PI O, who was wearing a Jackie Howe singlet. He was called up to read and I recall there was a lot of shouting involved with his delivery. I slurped wine, chain-smoked and waited for my call to the podium. Everyone seemed to be getting called up to read – everyone, of course, except me.

I riffled through my poems, selecting which ones I would read when my name was finally called. But after a while it became clear I was being ignored, and the more ignored I was, the more I drank. I polished off the whole carafe and ordered another for the table, and polished that off too in short order. Poet after poet got up to puke out their innermost feelings as I sat there fuming, wallowing in self-pity and an alcohol-induced funk. The poets were all a blur by now because the wine had gone to my head and the room swam.

'I think you've had enough,' said the guy next to me when he sat down after his reading.

'Christ, have I had enough!' I yelled. 'Whatever happened to the Aussie concept of a fair go? I've been sitting here listening to you bastards all night and I have to say I have never heard a bigger load of shite in all my life! If that's poetry, you can shove your poetry up your arse!'

There were blank looks all around. I had obviously fulfilled their expectations as the uncouth Queenslander out of his depth in the Big Smoke, but at that stage I couldn't have cared less. I did my best at storming out of there, and wandered the streets of King Cross for a while trying to cool down, poems clutched to my chest. I ended up in the notorious Bourbon & Beefsteak Bar later that night, and woke up the next morning on the cool, tiled floor of the loo back at my aunt and uncle's. Lord knows how I got there . . .

But a few months later my night of shame was forgotten when my poem, 'Night Ride Revisited', was accepted by Les and eventually published in *Poetry Australia*. When I got a copy of that edition in my hot little hand, I believed for a moment that I had been redeemed and that what Rod had once said was true. 'Poetry is God.'

The Pope *Will* Be Pleased

There was an audible sigh from behind the grate in the cramped confessional. I had been spilling my guts for about an hour and still felt I had a way to go, but the priest was obviously tiring.

'I think that's enough, my son,' he said, interrupting me. There was definitely a hint of exasperation in his voice.

'But, Father, I haven't finished with coveting yet,' I said. 'I really do want to give a full and frank confession.'

'Yes, I'm sure you do, but we've covered quite a lot of ground already and you can take it from me that you're coming in at the lower end of the scale in the sinning department. I really wonder how you can remember sins you committed when you were only two years old?'

'I have a frighteningly good memory,' I assured him. 'This is unfortunate, really, because when you can remember everything it gives you a lot to regret. And a lot to repent.'

There was a pregnant pause followed by what sounded

like the stifling of a yawn. But I pushed on with the business at hand. I mean, I wanted to get my money's worth since I was signing up to be a full-time Catholic and was determined to be accepted on legitimate grounds, which meant a comprehensive unburdening of myself via the sacrament of confession, or 'reconciliation' as they prefer it nowadays. I had my head bowed as I knelt in contrition, coughing up my litany of transgressions. I looked up again a few minutes later to see the priest behind the grate checking his watch. He sighed.

'And, Father, that's it, I'm done,' I said with a final flourish, pleased with my thoroughness and ready to have the slate wiped clean after a couple of decades' worth of utterly human foibles. Once this was behind me I would be ready for baptism and would then be a fully-fledged, spiritually paid-up, card-carrying member of the Holy Roman Catholic Church. I had dabbled with other denominations during my pilgrim's progress, it was true, but always found them wanting, and after much soul-searching had decided to go with the original and the best. (What was that motto the Commonwealth Bank used to have — 'Get with the strength'?)

This was the culmination of an extended dark night of the soul, one that had been going on for years. It had been kindled in the confusion of my student days, when I was what my father referred to as 'a crazy, mixed-up kid'. I think I can even pinpoint the time when this particular strand of what was to become an almost continuous existential crisis started to work up a proper head of steam. It was on a cold foggy winter's night in Toowoomba in 1976.

I was just emerging from my surfie hippie phase at the time and, being displaced from home and the beach, I guess I was feeling a bit unsettled, a bit vulnerable. As a first-year journalism student at the Darling Downs Institute of Advanced Education – as appropriate a name for an asylum as any – I was a student in the Arts faculty, and anyone involved in the Arts faculty was expected to behave strangely, even though the journalism students were regarded as squares by the hardcore arty farts. After a few months of excruciatingly boring lectures and exceedingly wild parties, my mental state was even more fragile. Passively smoking about 10 spliffs a day around the house – a dilapidated slum dwelling I shared with a dysfunctional group of fellow students in an unfashionable street – wasn't helping my psychological equilibrium. Nor was my diet, which consisted largely of toasted sandwiches, beer, cask wine, coffee and cigarettes. When the sandwich fillings ran out, as they often did, I resorted to eating butter and sugar sandwiches for dinner. In other words, I was wired, and becoming more so every day.

One foggy night we were all sitting around the house freezing and listening to John Lennon's album 'Shaved Fish' over and over again, as you tend to do when on the Bob Marley smoking cure. Two of my housemates, Ian and Steve, decided to be adventurous and cook up a soup utilising the gold-top magic mushrooms they had scored from someone at college that day. They created a foul-smelling broth – the rest of us passed on it (I have never been a fan of fungi, let alone the hallucinogenic kind) – then drank it and proceeded to start behaving like extras from *One Flew Over The Cuckoo's Nest*. Which was amusing for a few minutes but soon became tiresome, so I left them to it and went to my room, wrapped myself in some blankets and tried to read a book, but passed out soon afterwards. Later that evening one of the girls who also shared the house came and roused me from a dead sleep.

'I think we've got a problem,' she said.

'What sort of a problem?' I said, rubbing my eyes.

'Well, Ian and Steve went running, screaming, into the fog about an hour ago and they haven't come back. Since they are both tripping off their scones, I'm quite concerned.'

'So two have now flown over the cuckoo's nest,' I said.

'Huh?'

So I went out into the chilly, dark, dank night to search for them. It was a real pea-souper out there and a bit spooky. There was a vast park across the road and I did a sweep of it, searching for the escaped loonies. I wandered farther afield, into the streets and lanes nearby. It was even darker now, and the street lamps were mere smudges of light high above me. I crossed myself for protection, against whatever spooks hid in the mist — which was weird, because I wasn't Catholic, yet. My father's family had been, although most of them were well and truly lapsed. My father reckoned he'd give it the flick after being beaten by the Christian Brothers at boarding school in Hong Kong when he was a boy. He reckoned he was done with the Church from that moment on, although his youngest brother, my uncle Cyril, remained a practising Catholic, the most devout of all the Browns, throughout his life.

I could understand my dad's point of view, but I felt a family tradition had been broken. I was baptised in a Presbyterian church because my mother's family were Protestants, and I did go to Sunday School for a little while, but by the time I started primary school, religion was off the agenda in our family. Still, I had retained a vague interest, and sometimes flicked through a Bible I had been given as a child. I felt some attachment to Christianity and had always felt jealous of a childhood friend who used to cross himself at assembly at the end of the Lord's Prayer. I'd always wanted to do that, too.

I felt better after crossing myself now, and as I wandered around in the dark – a fool looking for two other fools – I started to wonder why I imagined crossing myself could protect me. I thought I must believe in it if it made me feel better and I guess I felt that – it sounds silly – I kind of felt that Jesus would protect me. This set me thinking – not that I hadn't been thinking already. Mostly, all I ever did was think at that stage of my life, in between bouts of carousing. Occasionally I would write as well as think, mainly mawkish poems pondering the great questions of existence. But mostly I thought, because it was easier than actually doing anything.

So there I was, wandering in the fog now, wondering about the meaning of life and what to do about it. I felt an imperative to act in some way to solve my existential angst, but I wasn't quite sure how. I crossed myself again to ward off the nasties of the night and continued to search for my friends, who were not only off their tree but, as it turned out, up one when I eventually found them. They were both perched on a sturdy lower branch, hooting like owls. This made me glad I had vowed never to engage in the taking of hallucinogens, because intuition told me that if I did, I would just go up and never come down. Anyway, I coaxed them down, which wasn't easy, and led them back home. They hooted all the way. Poor buggers, I thought. I didn't want to end up like that, although I feared I too was going a bit batty living on bad food, in penury, and with drug-crazed companions who spent more time stoned than straight. I craved something deeper.

In the weeks following this bizarre incident I stepped up my spiritual readings and ponderings. I had already dabbled in the field and had been very impressed with Malcolm Muggeridge's book, *Something Beautiful for God*, which was about Mother Teresa of Calcutta. The fact that he was a well-known broadcaster gave his religious leanings extra credibility as far as I was concerned. I had been a C S Lewis fan since childhood and had also read some of his theological works – including *Mere Christianity* – and was much taken with some of his ideas and his plain, reasonable prose. The fact that I loved his Narnia chronicles and an obscure science fiction trilogy of his that I'd read as a teenager (*Out of The Silent Planet*, *Perelandra* and *That Hideous Strength*) lent something more to his Christian writings. Not that Lewis was as fashionable then as he is now. In fact, nobody I knew was reading any such thing, so I kept this particular strand of my literary browsing largely under my hat. The books that students back then were into was stuff by Hermann Hesse,

Richard Brautigan and Hunter S Thompson, not theological musings by some fuddy-duddy Oxford don. I also read Lewis's *The Screwtape Letters*, basically a satirical but pointed book of letters from one devil to another on matters pertaining to tempting humans into sin. The problem of evil and the existence, or not, of Satan became something of a mild obsession.

In retrospect my behaviour back then seems quite nutty, even a tad psychotic. I took to going on long walks at night trying to work it all out – evil, suffering, the whole kit and caboodle of life. In the dark, often foggy, back streets of the quiet, conservative western suburbs of Toowoomba, I challenged Beelzebub to come out and face me like a man, and I would denounce him and all his works – which covered quite a lot of territory. I guess I was basing my mad meanderings and confrontations with the dark one on the gospel descriptions of Jesus being taunted and tempted during his stint in the wilderness, when he ultimately rejected Satan and all the wicked ways of the world. While modelling myself on that wasn't the sort of behaviour one would expect of a 19-year-old surfie, my housemates tolerated it, even if they did look askance at me from time to time. The fact that I hadn't eaten a decent meal for months was probably having some sort of effect on me. Besides the sugar sandwiches and occasional hamburger, my diet consisted of coffee, Mars bars, and vanilla slices from the refectory when I was at college. My blood sugar dipped and dived regularly, and I attended to that with more sugar and caffeine. So now that I look back at it, my crisis was probably caused by little more than some sort of nutritional deficiency. I'm recounting these sad dietary habits because I think they might help explain the precarious state of my constitution and, correspondingly, my state of mind. That might be the empirical assessment, at least.

But I was young and naïve and full of questions about the world, and in my naïveté I figured my elders might know a bit more about all this than I did. So I took to calling on – some might say pestering – the college chaplain on a weekly basis and engaged him, occasionally against his will, it seemed, in deep and meaningfuls about aspects of Christianity, and in particular the veracity of the gospels. Our conversations never really resolved much, though, and I could tell that I tried his patience much of the time because he obviously had a fairly conservative approach to his religion.

'The problem is that the Bible is full of contradictions,' I said to him one day.

He shook his head firmly, being the evangelical, Bible-believing kind of guy that he was. 'Oh my word, no, the Bible is very clear on everything,' he said. 'The Bible is unimpeachable as the word of God. We take it on faith that it is His word, verbatim, and the will of the Creator is outlined very clearly in Holy Scripture.'

'But when it says that those who are last shall then be first, and that those who are first shall then be last ... don't you find that confusing?'

'Not at all,' he insisted, holding his big, floppy Bible in his lap.

'And Jesus says peacemakers are blessed, and yet he goes into the temple and kicks shit out of the joint, tips over all the money-lenders' stalls and gives them a boot up the bum for good measure. Don't you find that, well, a bit ambiguous? I know I do.'

'There is no ambiguity in Scripture,' he insisted again, holding firm. 'Faith reveals the truth in Scripture to those who will hear it.'

'As in, "let those who have ears hear"?' I said. 'Although on the other hand, if you didn't have ears and couldn't hear it might not necessarily be your fault. You might have leprosy or something.'

He looked troubled, and I could see the word 'vexation' forming in his brain. 'Well, I'm afraid we'll have to wind up there for today,' he said. 'I have someone else to see, so we'll continue this some other time.'

Eventually, however, the appointments with the chaplain dried up, because he seemed to get very busy in the following weeks and I couldn't get to see him. It's not a nice feeling when a clergyman drops you: I had a touch of the 'it's not you, it's me's' after that, and felt that maybe I was unworthy. But luckily there was a glimmer of hope on the horizon and a more accepting religious mentor not far around the corner.

On one of my last visits to the chaplaincy I had picked up a magazine called *The Word* – a publication put out by the Divine Word Missionaries, a Catholic order that helped people in third world countries. I was entering the altruistic and messianic stage of my religious delusion by now, and the idea of going out into the world and doing good, saving people and redeeming humanity appealed to me. The seeds of this idea had been sown when I'd read Muggeridge's book about Mother Teresa. I had ideas above my station. Using a coupon in the magazine, I wrote away asking for more information, thinking I might like to get involved somewhere, somehow. I didn't tell them at this stage that I wasn't Catholic. I got a nice letter back from Father Bill Burt, the head of the order in Australia at the time, explaining the work they did and telling me that if I wanted to find out about the order I was welcome to visit them. Coincidentally, their seminary was a beautiful and historic mansion on a hill at Marburg, halfway between Toowoomba and the Gold Coast. I knew the spot — you can see it from the highway — and had often wondered what went on there when I was driving by. Or hitchhiking past, as was often the case in those days. I subscribed to *The Word* magazine shortly afterwards, and wrote back to Father Bill telling him that I would come and visit one day. This sparked an occasional correspondence between us, particularly since Father Bill was keen on the literary life. His interest helped me get over being so callously jilted by the college chaplain.

I was living two different lives at this time — my Gold Coast surfie life, which had been on hold, and my serious, angst-ridden poet-student-spiritual seeker life. They were separated by distance and shaped by geography and my daily surrounds. In my summer holidays I was back on the Gold Coast, surfing and distracted by the Christmas party scene, so my spiritual odyssey was on hold for a while. It seemed compartmentalised as part of my Toowoomba life, a separate entity, particularly when the waves were good and the sun was shining. But when I started my second year of college, the quest was back on the agenda. Kerry Drysdale, a schoolmate who had been a seminarian in Brisbane for a year but had left to pursue art, moved into a new share-house I had shifted to, and that got me going on the Catholic stuff again. He didn't talk much about his stint in the seminary but I got the feeling he had enjoyed the monastic life there only up to a point. He was disappointed he'd dropped out but felt he would probably serve God better as a lay person. He was still adjusting to being in the wide world again and on a campus where girls outnumbered boys. He encouraged me to go to Mass with him, and I got to like the ritual and formality of the service. The Catholic thing had a whiff of literary credibility about it too, I felt. There were, of course, stellar literary models such as Graham Greene and Evelyn Waugh to go on. And then two of Australia's greatest poets, Bruce Dawe and Les Murray — who were, as you know, fast becoming personal friends of mine — were practising Catholics.

As a young and very impressionable poet, I thought this Catholic malarky might be the go. I'd be in good company and I'd always had an ascetic side — even though that side fluctuated wildly at college, where I would read the gospels and crank out faux metaphysical doggerel, then go on a party jag that lasted a week. Eventually, after too much partying and too little study, I decided to drop out of college.

My constitution had suffered from the dissolute lifestyle, and I went back to the Gold Coast. Even though I had elected to leave Toowoomba, I felt I had failed by throwing it in – which served to heighten my existential angst.

Instead of mooching around surfing, which I'd planned to do pretty much full-time, I got a job – courtesy of my dad, who collared me and marched me to the interview. But being tied to a desk wasn't much of a stimulant after what I'd been up to, so in my restlessness I continued my religious browsing.

I noticed an ad in *The Catholic Leader* for a correspondence course that was supposed to prepare you for becoming a Catholic. It was over something like three months, and basically the Church would just send you brochures which would set you up with all you needed to know to become a member of the one true church. I wrote to Father Bill and told him about all this, hoping he'd be impressed. When I signed up for the course I got a very enthusiastic response to my enquiry. Thereafter the brochures lobbed in regularly. The course was fairly rudimentary, starting with a historical context that proved, of course, that the Catholic Church was the one true church, in case I hadn't realised that already. Then, brochure by brochure, I was taken through the tenets of the faith, what Catholics believe, and the various sacraments and how they fitted into the spiritual life of a Catholic. The ritualistic approach appealed to me, and the brochures explained it all very clearly, which helped. I would pore over the material in my room at night, puffing on the pipe which was part of my affectation at the time. Looking back on it, I should have had a smoking jacket to complete the image, but mostly I just wore an old tartan gown.

One of the reasons I wanted to become a Catholic was that I had a vague fantasy about becoming a priest. Kerry, my ex-seminarian friend, had made it sound pretty romantic. I hadn't thought it out at that stage – the celibacy, the hard work, the commitment – but just fancied the notion of wearing the gear, feeling holy and saving the world. When I wrote to Father Bill and told him I was studying to become a Catholic via mail-order brochures, he sounded impressed, even a little excited, and invited me to visit the Divine Word seminarians while they were on retreat at Marburg. I was thrilled! Maybe some of it would rub off and I would find a vocation with them. Anything seemed possible. I didn't know what to expect, but it sounded much more glamorous than writing ads for a radio station, which was how I'd been filling my time when I wasn't busy with the correspondence course.

So one weekend I pointed my trusty Falcon 500 westwards and lobbed into Marburg. The seminary building and grounds were grand and impressive, though it felt more like a country club than a seminary at first. I was warmly welcomed by Father Bill and introduced to the seminarians, who seemed like a pretty ordinary bunch of guys. They were mainly in their twenties and didn't have halos hovering above their heads or anything. I'm not sure what I expected – bearded ascetics with pronounced auras, perhaps? – but they all seemed like plain, friendly blokes not all that different from me. I went to Mass with them in the small chapel there, and there was a palpable feeling of joy and fellowship – something that's talked about a lot at various churches, but not always present. Someone played a guitar, very softly, while Father Bill gave a homily about faith. As the Scripture says, if you have faith even as small as a mustard seed, it will be effective. Mustard seeds were handed out for effect, and they sure are pretty bloody small: I dropped mine almost as soon as it hit the palm of my hand, and then hoped desperately it wasn't a Sign.

In the evening I sat in the living room and chatted with Father Bill over a couple of glasses of port. Very civilised seminary, this, I thought. We chatted about the order's work, which included missionary work all around the world, primarily giving practical help to communities in Third World countries by demonstrating the love of God in action. There was an evangelistic agenda too, but this was subtle and promoted more by action than by aggressive proselytising, which appealed to me. Mostly, though, we chatted about literature. He was a big reader, and very keen on Lawrence Durrell in particular. He urged me to read the famous *Alexandria Quartet*, something I've always meant to do since but have never quite got around to.

That night I shared a room with a young seminarian who was into music – he had a cassette of the Rolling Stones playing quietly in the room – and behaved nothing like a future priest should, as far as I could tell.

'Do you really want to be a priest?' I asked him that night as we got ready for sleep.

'Well, my mother wants me to,' he answered.

'That's not really enough, though, I imagine, is it?'

'Probably not,' he said. 'I doubt if I will last, actually. I've already been getting into quite a bit of strife and this is just my first year.'

'What sort of strife?' I asked.

'Well, I smuggled a girl into my room one night.'

'Oh, I can see how that could be a problem when you're supposed to be celibate.'

'Yes, but nothing happened,' he said. 'We were just talking.'

'Yes, but we all know that talking can lead to sex. If you're lucky.'

'It didn't go down too well,' he said. 'Plus I've had a bit too much to drink on a few occasions and that hasn't exactly endeared me to the powers-that-be.'

'It is the priesthood you've signed up for, after all,' I said. 'It's not supposed to be easy, is it?' As I was saying this, I began to have serious doubts about my own suitability. No girls, no grog, lots of hard work – it didn't sound like a lot of fun, regardless of how worthy it might be.

'But it beats the hell out of working for a living,' he said. 'What about you?'

'Well, the idea sort of appeals to me,' I replied. 'Helping people seems like a good thing to do. But actually I'm not even Catholic . . . yet.' But I fully intended to become one – and sooner rather than later.

'What do you mean, *yet*?' he asked.

'Well, I'm doing a course.'

'What sort of course?'

'One of those correspondence courses they advertise in *The Catholic Leader*,' I said proudly.

'That's hilarious,' he said. 'I can't believe anyone actually responds to those ads.' He saw me look a bit crestfallen. 'But no, actually I think that's a good thing,' he backpedalled. 'I mean, if you're sincere and really want to become a Catholic, that's great. We sure as hell need new recruits.'

'I'm nearly finished the course, actually, so I think I'll be getting confirmed in the next few months.'

'Wonderful,' he said, turning out the light and then adding from the darkness, 'The Pope *will* be pleased.'

But after further self-examination, I didn't think I was made of the right stuff to join the priesthood, and while my weekend at Marburg was pleasant, I was convinced that I would be better off as a member of the laity. Which led me not long afterwards to my first confession and acceptance into the Catholic Church. I would become one of its most ambivalent adherents over the next few decades. The Pope might not be so pleased about *that*.

Clap if You Love Jesus

I was supposed to be writing crappy radio commercials, not reading the Mahatma's autobiography. But it was that time of the afternoon when the human spirit sags and needs chocolate, coffee or some other sort of inspiration to push through the doldrums. I pulled out my tatty, cloth-covered volume of *The Story of My Experiments With Truth* by Mohandas K Gandhi. I had bought it at an alternative bookshop the week before and was halfway through. While I was reading, someone said: 'It's the devil's work, you know.'

'What?' I asked, looking up, not sure if I had heard right.

'Yoga, it's the devil's work, sent to tempt a new generation.'

The proponent of this preposterous proclamation was Jeff, the production guy I worked with at 4GG, the Gold Coast's pre-eminent radio station at the time (the late Seventies). Religion wasn't a typical conversation-piece here because 'Double-G', as we called it, was a very secular place – a bastion of crass commercialism and a celebrity hotspot where, on any given day, you might run into Barry

Humphries or Sammy Davis Jnr in the hallway. In fact that very morning I had bumped into a star of stage, screen and kitchen – Bernard King, resplendent in a large, floppy, red hat.

'Oh, hellooooo,' he'd cooed. 'A new face . . . lovely. I'll keep my eye out for you.' I certainly hoped not.

The station manager, the charismatic former Melbourne disc jockey Barry Ferber, seemed to know every celebrity on the planet. That and the fact that we were on the fabulous Gold Coast made 4GG a pretty 'up' sort of place to work, with everyone swanning around in regulation floral shirts, perpetually smiling. Well, almost everyone.

I was a depressed young poet going through a spiritual crisis. And Jeff was a born-again Christian who couldn't keep his mouth shut about his beliefs. He had no problem with the perpetual smile, but his proselytising didn't fit into the GG scene too well. Jeff had interesting ideas, openly promoting masturbation above sex (what's wrong with both, I wanted to know), and lived on junk food and soft drink, certain that the salvation of his immortal soul meant his body was immune to the normal rules of physics. Given that he was pasty-faced with pimples and had rounded shoulders from slouching over a console his entire working life, I wasn't sure that God was living up to His part of the deal.

But Jeff had definitely found his truth – Jesus, Jesus and more bloody Jesus was all he talked about all day long. Not that I had a problem with Jesus: I had been reading the gospels on and off with some interest since my mid-teens and was now deep into my correspondence course for intending Catholics. But I hadn't taken my leap of faith quite yet and, frankly, I was kind of enjoying my temporary ambivalence about committing to any one faith. Meanwhile, I was devouring all manner of spiritual texts, trying to work out the meaning of life, as you do when you're 21 – which is why I was reading Gandhi.

'Gandhi' also happened to be a nickname of mine at the time. My father, a thick-set bloke to say the least, was puzzled by my svelte physique (he used to say I was 'built like a racing tadpole'), and had called me Gandhi when I started wearing little round glasses and prayer shirts. So I thought I'd read up on the guy, and took the book to work with me. It was my humble job to write scripts for the excruciating ads you would have heard on your car radio if you had been driving on the Gold Coast back in those days.

I worked in a room the size of a broom closet with a sliding door on either side. Advertising salesmen breezed in regularly, dumped their orders in my in-tray, and I would turn their scribbled briefs into 20-, 30- or 60-second commercials. Jeff would retrieve the finished scripts from another tray and take them into the recording studio, where the announcers – blokes with impossibly deep, enthusiastic voices – would read them out, accompanied by cheesy background music. There were ads for car dealerships, restaurants, electrical appliance stores and the vast, treeless canal estates that were proliferating at that time. Jeff would put the ads on cassettes, which then went into the studio. In between all that he'd harass me, like now, because he saw me reading something he thought looked suspicious.

'This book is not about yoga, it's about Gandhi,' I said.

'Is he a Christian?' he asked.

'He's dead,' I said. 'So it doesn't matter.'

'But was he saved before he died?' Jeff asked.

'Well, Gandhi said he was a Christian and a Muslim and a Buddhist,' I offered. 'He had all his bases covered, so I guess the answer is yes.'

'Impossible,' said Jeff. 'No-one can get to God save through the Son.' He often spoke in this lofty, Scriptural manner, which was something of an anachronism considering where we lived and worked. This was, after all, the land of hedonism – a place where every day was a sunny day and radio announcers refrained from talking about the rain on inclement days for fear it would turn the tourists off. Jeff and I seemed the only ones concerned with anything beyond the temporal.

I was there, I felt, by accident. After dropping out of college I'd spent months moping around the house watching telly and writing poetry, though not at the same time. My father kept suggesting I get a job, and when he realised I wasn't going to do anything about that myself, he got one for me. He knew Barry Ferber, had spoken to him about his unemployed son, and suggested I go see the radio boss forthwith. During my interview with Barry I hoped to dissuade him from hiring me, but unfortunately he took a shine to me. Next thing I knew, I was sitting in the world's smallest office staring at the filing cabinets, wondering where I'd gone wrong.

Working on the theory that it takes one to know one, Jeff had soon zeroed in on me as a kindred spirit. Nobody else in the station seemed quite on his wavelength, but he thought I was — though I was also something of a challenge for him. He considered poetry, which I tapped out on my huge typewriter between ads, spiritually dangerous, and was constantly shaking his head over my reading matter. *Jonathan Livingston Seagull* would have been Beelzebub's work to Jeff. There was only one book for him and you can guess what it was.

'But Jesus and Gandhi had a lot in common, actually,' I tried to reason with him.

'Don't even say that, amen,' he said. 'Praise Jesus.' He punctuated his conversation with evangelical declamations, waving his arms in the air.

'Gandhi was a man of peace in the same way Jesus was,' I tried.

'"Man of peace"? Jesus was the *prince* of peace,' Jeff said. 'The light of the world, the very Son of God!' He was starting to rant.

'Keep your voice down,' I said. 'Anyway, I've got some ads to write.'

Before getting back to work, I opened my drawer and took out a bottle of Mylanta, the antacid medicine I'd been virtually living on since being diagnosed with the beginnings of a duodenal ulcer. This was apparently the result of my wayward dietary practices as a student, and had been diagnosed by the family GP, who suggested it also had a lot to do with the fact that I was a natural worrier. I had tried various tablets to no avail and was now on a strict diet consisting, if I recall correctly, of yoghurt, cracker biscuits, cottage cheese, herbal tea and not much else — except, of course, the Mylanta. I took a swig of the foul liquid every so often to keep the ulcer pain at bay, gagging in the process.

'What is that stuff?' Jeff asked. He was still lurking.

'Oh, just something for my ulcer,' I said.

'Your ulcer?' he said, astonished. '*Your ulcer*! You're too young to have an ulcer.'

'Apparently not.'

'Praise the Lord . . . Jesus heals ulcers,' he said. 'Jesus heals everything. You just have to ask and ye shall receive, knock and the door shall be open unto you . . . '

He was off again, but I was saved from another sermon by Tony, one of the advertising reps, who barged into the room and shoved a piece of paper in front of me. 'Can you have this done in an hour?' he asked, but it was more of a demand really. 'That's if Reverend Jeff here will leave you alone so you can get on with it.'

'Very funny,' said Jeff. 'But mock not the Lord our God.'

'Why not?' snapped Tony. 'He's been mocking me for 50-odd years now. If he can dish it out, surely he can take it too.'

That sent Jeff from the room, promising to be back. He and I had unfinished business, he reckoned. I wiped the white Mylanta moustache from my upper lip, put the book away and started to hammer out another inanity while the station's easy-listening music oozed from the wall microphone behind me. It was the overripe, cheesy sound of

Clap if You Love Jesus

'Reminiscing' by The Little River Band — and boy, did I wish they would give it a break. I never could stand schmaltz like that, but listening to it eight hours a day was compulsory here at fun central, 4GG.

The days, lived out to the tunes of LRB, Air Supply and others, sometimes seemed endless there in my broom closet, and it was scribbling poetry and reading which got me through, along with practical jokes. Sometimes Jeff and I would raid the props department for laughs. Despite often managing to sound like John the Baptist, the guy did have a sense of humour. We'd dig stuff out of the props box — wigs, fake ears, clown noses, Dracula teeth (God knows what they used this stuff for) — and wear them, me at my desk, he in the production studio, waiting for the double-takes from our colleagues when they came along. It was pretty puerile but it amused us.

At home in the evenings I wrote endless poems about the whys and wherefores of existence and read other spiritually-inclined books by the likes of Teilhard de Chardin and Dietrich Bonhoeffer. Not exactly light-hearted stuff, but that was my mood.

In stark contrast, by day I cranked out ads and the occasional jingle (I once wrote a really dreadful one which was performed by the country singer Lee Conway) and snacked on Ryvitas and yoghurt. I really wanted to get rid of the intermittent pain in my guts and I did wonder why the Creator of the Universe had decided to visit such an affliction on me . . . poor me!

I tried not to talk too much about this to Jeff, though,

who was still popping into my office regularly to drop off pamphlets for his Pentecostal church and deliver mini-sermons. By now I was busy re-reading T S Eliot's poems – probably not the sort of thing you need when you're a bit depressed and have a tummy ache. I had typed bits of poems, cut them out and stuck them onto my desk with sticky tape.

Jeff was trying to read one of them upside down from the other side of my desk. ' "I should have been a pair of ragged claws scuttling across the floors of silent seas"?' he intoned. 'What the heck does that mean?'

'It's a poetic metaphor for Eliot's existential disassociation,' I said.

'He wouldn't have an eggertenshal whatchamacallit if he had Jesus in his heart,' Jeff replied.

'Well, he was quite religious later in his life and was a regular churchgoer,' I protested.

'Yes, but there are churches and churches,' he said with his usual brilliance. 'What about you, are you going to church?'

'I go to Mass now and then,' I said.

'You want to come to a real, spirit-filled church,' he said. 'Hey, there's a crusade and mass healing service on this weekend that I'm going to. Why don't you come along? You can cure that ulcer and you won't have to drink any more of that horrible white goo you've been swigging.'

'I'm pretty busy this weekend,' I said.

'Too busy for God?'

'Well, I'm sure He's pretty busy too.'

Jeff shook his head. 'I think you should come along and

see what happens,' he said, and he badgered me about it for the next couple of days. Eventually I caved in and said I would go with him. The truth is, I was curious, and deep down wondered whether there was a chance that I might experience something miraculous. What did I have to lose? I'd never been to a Pentecostal service but had seen some on television, and they seemed a bit wacky and simplistic to me. I favoured a more complex, mystical approach, which was probably why I had an ulcer. But it wouldn't hurt to give the holy rollers a shot, would it?

So I agreed to meet Jeff outside the Miami State High School hall, where a Christian rally was being held that Saturday night. When I'd gone to school there it was an educational facility where half the student body majored in surfing and dope smoking. I was glad to escape the place and hadn't been back since then, so it was weird being in these school grounds again, milling outside the hall where we used to have assembly. I noticed a few familiar faces in the crowd, including a couple of guys I knew from the beach. Born-again Christianity had made some inroads into the surfing scene at the time and had probably saved a few lives by turning young people away from drugs and into tiresome God-botherers instead. For a few years there had even been a Christian board riders' club, which was always out for new converts. If you saw one of those guys walking down the beach, you'd turn and walk in the opposite direction. A guy I knew from school who'd become a member spotted me now, came over and pumped my hand.

'Good to see ya here,' he gushed. 'Amen, hallelujah.'

'Yeah, good to be here,' I said gingerly.

'Yeah, he's in the right place, amen,' said Jeff as we all streamed inside and took our seats in the darkened hall. A little while later, some abysmal gospel rock music started up, a spotlight hit the stage, and into it walked a fat bloke in a three-piece suit. Not exactly Gold Coast casual wear. He carried a microphone, which he tossed from hand to hand for a bit, like Tom Jones. Then he put it too close to his mouth and for a moment I thought he was going to sing 'The Green Green Grass of Home', but instead he shouted: 'Do ya love Jesus?!' There was a mild hubbub and sporadic shouts of 'Yes!' and 'Amen!'

'I said, do you really love Jesus?!' he shouted again, louder this time and with a bit of reverberation added by the sound guy. The crowd became more enthusiastic now. Jeff was nudging me to get involved but I have never been prone to emotional ejaculations.

'Well that's grand. So let's hear it for the Lord then!' the preacher urged. 'Come on, everybody, clap if ya love Jesus. I say clap if ya love Jesus.' His voice had a distinct American twang; actually, he sounded a bit like the Looney Tunes rooster, Foghorn Leghorn.

'Where is this guy from?' I asked Jeff, who was very excited and applauding madly.

'Dalby, amen,' he said.

After establishing that everyone did in fact love Jesus, the preacher — I think his name was Pastor Ray — started to tell us about how he'd come to the Lord. He had been a bikie in his past life, a profaner and a wicked defiler of women; a sinner who drank and cussed and embraced evil, and a man whose heart was full of hate. It sounded like he'd been busy and had plenty of fun, too. But then he met Jesus one day on a long, lonely stretch of highway in the Darling Downs, his own road to Damascus. That turned his life around, and since then he'd been to Bible college in America, where they had obviously furnished him with a burning fundamentalist belief and turned him into a crushing bore with a bad American accent.

'The Lord said to me, "Feed my sheep"!' he shouted again, obviously confusing himself with the Son of God. 'He said to me, "Ray, go among your people and anoint them with the Holy Spirit. Turn them away from the devil as you were turned away. Bring faith, hope and healing to them in the name of Jesus. In the name of Jesus!" Now let us pray, brothers and sisters.' He bowed his head.

'Pretty impressive,' said Jeff, who was now holding his hands above his head and starting to sway.

'Pretty derivative,' I said.

After praying a bit, Pastor Ray – whose accent lapsed occasionally, revealing flashes of broad Strine – gave us some more blarney about his mission to the people of the Darling Downs, which he made sound like some sort of Sodom and Gomorrah. He'd turned some prostitutes there away from their wicked ways, like veritable Mary Magdalenes. I wasn't aware they even had prostitutes on the Darling Downs.

'And I said to them, "Come down out of that house of sin, repent now and praise the Lord",' he said with gravity.

'And they came down weeping and we prayed, and they received the Holy Spirit and we gave praise to the Lord Jesus Christ for his infinite mercy.'

Talk about a corny script.

'Pretty amazing, don't you think?' said Jeff, apparently awestruck.

'Yeah,' I said. 'I went to college in Toowoomba for a year-and-a-half and I never saw one hooker the whole time.'

He looked at me. Then everyone started jumping up and down as Pastor Ray declared that the Holy Spirit had entered the hall. With his mouth on the microphone now — contravening health and safety standards, I was sure — he was making 'whooshing' sound effects to indicate that the Holy Spirit was moving around the hall and over the audience like some dervish. It sounded more like waves crashing on a beach to me, but what do I know?

Then he started calling for people to come forward and accept Jesus as their 'personal Lord and Saviour' and receive a healing from him. As he did so, various minions rushed up and down the rows passing along collection plates, which were being filled to the brim. It was brilliant strategic fundraising, striking when everyone was in a lather. People were forking over $20 notes with abandon, and I felt a bit cheap just tossing in some shrapnel, but there was no way I was investing my hard-earned money. Surely God is free . . .

As the money was being collected, people began rushing to the stage and lining up. Pastor Ray, still making whooshing sounds, laid his hands on the foreheads of the faithful. Two assistants then pushed these people to the floor, where they writhed and twitched. They call it 'slain in spirit', I think, and it really is very silly.

'Now's your chance,' said Jeff, so I went down the aisle and lined up with everyone else because it would have caused trouble if I hadn't. I was more curious than anything, but my rumbling tummy suggested another ulcer attack coming on, so I thought I'd test Pastor Ray's powers. I might as well get some value for the money I'd put in the collection plate. Before I knew it I had ascended the stage, virtually dragged up there by the henchmen, and Pastor Ray was whispering in my ear. 'What is your problem, brother?'

'Where to start . . . ' I said. 'Um, I've got an ulcer.'

'Uh, huh,' he said. 'Uh, huh. Well, we're going to call on the Holy Spirit to loose this ulcer, to banish it from your body and to make you whole as you accept Jesus Christ as your personal Lord and Saviour.'

Conditions always apply, don't they?

I nodded half-heartedly and he slapped a large clammy paw on my forehead while his henchmen pulled at my shoulders from behind, trying to drag me down onto the stage, where several people now lay flip-flopping like fish out of water. I fought against them, so Pastor Ray pushed harder against my forehead. Eventually they got me to my knees, which was as far as I would go. They left me kneeling there and quickly moved on to the next person. I stood up immediately, feeling very embarrassed, and virtually ran back to my seat. It was weird, particularly in light of the fact that the last time I'd been on that stage I was playing a knight in the musical *Camelot*.

'Amazing,' said Jeff. 'You're healed!'

'Am I? I don't feel any different.'

'But you must,' he insisted. 'There's a powerful healing here tonight.'

'There's a powerful something,' I said.

The service lasted an hour-and-a-half in all, and by the end of it I was, you might say, sceptical about evangelical Christianity. But when you're young, the more bizarre things are, the more they tend to appeal to you. Pastor Ray could have been a character out of the rock opera *Tommy*, I thought. All the characters in that show seemed hyper-real, caricatures of caricatures, although I do recall being stoned out of my mind when I saw it, so I may have been doing the good pastor a disservice. But he did revel in his performance, which may have been a lot more palatable if the soundtrack had consisted of music by The Who instead of the flaky rock outfit that was banging out the Jesus tunes on this night. As for the healing power . . . well, that didn't seem to take because I still had a gut ache when I got home. I wondered: if God could heal, why hadn't He healed me? Was I so unworthy?

At work, Jeff seemed surprised to find me still scoffing Mylanta. He blamed me for the fact that the hocus-pocus hadn't worked. I was a resister, he suggested, whose head was too full of wicked ideas gleaned from modern literature and Eastern philosophy for faith to take hold properly.

Somehow Jeff talked me into attending a prayer breakfast with him a few weeks later. It was held at a function centre in Nerang, of all places, which was little more than a hamlet back then. It was a scary affair where glossolalia – talking in tongues – was on the menu. The idea does have a Biblical basis, deriving from an incident in the Book of Acts when, on the Day of Pentecost, the Paraclete (the Holy Spirit) had the apostles and their close companions jabbering away in various tongues, strange tongues. They were understood by everyone because everyone imagined they heard them talking in their own lingo. The born-agains had taken this practice up big-time, but the combined effect of everyone doing it sounded like a crowd of people all saying 'birdie num num' together.

The bloke next to me seemed particularly adept, and was running off at the mouth something shocking. He was a tall, swarthy dude, unlike the rest of the assembly, who were all Anglo and looked like Mormons. Anyway, we got chatting – his name was Carlos, he had migrated here from Central America, and he worked as a landscape gardener. He had a gentle way about him and seemed much less extreme than the others, so I was kind of glad to be next to him. I had Jeff on the other side of me and he was babbling away unintelligibly. He sounded more like he was being taken over by a parakeet than the Paraclete.

This whole business of talking in tongues actually scared the hell out of me. There was way too much abandon involved for a control freak like me. It was weird, and supposedly a gift from the Holy Spirit; but what the unintelligible gibbering going on around me had to do with all that, I don't know. It sounded like 'The Goon Show' played backward. And how did they know they were all channelling the Holy Spirit and not some other, far less savoury entity? I'm never very good in the mornings, and this was all a bit much for me at breakfast.

Back at work, the boss seemed a bit concerned about my friendship with Jeff, who he obviously thought was a fruitcake. He stuck his head into my cupboard one day to see how I was going.

'You're not going to God too, are you?' he asked.

'Come in, my son, and I'll tell you,' I jested.

'Very funny,' he said. 'I don't want your father blaming me if you turn all religious on us. Now write some more bloody ads, will you, or none of us will get paid.'

Jeff cooled off on the proselytising for a few weeks, but he couldn't help himself and started in on me again eventually – probably because I was the only person in the building who didn't tell him to 'fuck off' when he started talking about Jesus.

He was convinced that I needed to give the Lord another crack at fixing my tummy trouble. In other words, he wanted me to go to another healing service with him.

'I've tried and failed miserably,' I said.

'But all you need is faith as big as a mustard seed,' he said.

'Oh, don't mention mustard,' I said, gripping my belly. 'Anyway, I don't even know what a mustard seed looks like,' I lied.

'But I'm convinced that if you give God a go, He will heal you,' he said quite earnestly. 'I think you should come and meet Reverend Jim at Broadbeach. You haven't been to one of his services before, have you?'

'No I have not,' I said.

'There's a very powerful healing force working through him lately,' he said. 'The Holy Spirit has really anointed him. Come with me on Sunday night?'

I weakened – my social life was non-existent at this stage – and said I'd give it one last go. I went to pick Jeff up at his flat in Surfers Paradise that Sunday evening. He was just finishing his dinner: doughnuts and Coke.

'That stuff will kill you,' I said.

'We all die eventually,' he said. 'And man does not live by bread alone.'

'Nor bloody doughnuts,' I said.

He was convinced that as long as he read his Bible, went to church regularly and abstained from extramarital sexual intercourse, he would be fine; that God would take care of the rest, including, presumably, his diabetes.

We drove down to Broadbeach, where the service was happening underneath a big old beach house just a block from the dunes. This was familiar territory because I'd spent my late teens surfing and partying around here, but I certainly didn't know of any churches under houses. Lots of bong sessions, but no churches.

The holy rollers were in full swing with a small rock band – the neighbours must have been thrilled. We got out of the car and I followed Jeff into the space under the house, where about 20 or 30 people were gathered, hands uplifted, eyes closed, praising the Lord big-time. Reverend Jim – I figured the guy with the Old Testament beard had to be him – had an electric guitar slung around his neck. It rested nicely on his pot belly and he was plucking at it and chanting something into a microphone in front of him. It sounded like the recipe for a very complicated curry, but of course he was talking in tongues. It was gibberish, but everyone seemed to be getting off on it, convinced it was proof that the Holy Spirit had descended from above and was now running the proceedings.

'Welcome, brothers, welcome,' Reverend Jim said as we came in. 'In the name of JESSSUUUUSSSSS.' He was doing that whooshing thing with the microphone – these preachers must learn it at Bible College: 'Holy Spirit arriving microphone technique 101'.

'Find a seat and let's give glory to God,' he said to us and then started plucking his guitar, leading the congregation in a hymn.

'This time I'm sure it will work for you,' Jeff said. 'I can just feel the spirit here.' He started stamping his feet and clapping then, like the other loonies. Meanwhile, Reverend Jim and his flock finished murdering the hymn – whatever it was, I certainly didn't recognise it – and he started his sermon, which was a series of Biblical clichés punctuated by warnings of doom and gloom.

'For the time is upon us, brothers and sisters!' he warned. 'The end time. Old men will dream dreams and young men will see visions and there will be wars and rumours of war throughout the world. And Satan will rise in the form of a man and he will display the mark of the beast upon his forehead and his rise will usher in the beginning of the end.' He seemed happy about this.

'Nothing like a bit of positive thinking,' I muttered. The crowd was busy going 'amen' and 'praise the Lord' and 'yes, Jesus, yes!'. I started thinking about leaving even though I'd only just arrived, but I was trapped like a rat.

Eventually there was a lull in the proceedings while Reverend Jim took a few sips of water (or was it gin?) and announced that the healing would commence. 'And I can feel there are some among us tonight who need a healing very badly,' he said, closing his eyes and holding the microphone close to his mouth. 'And I know that the Holy Spirit is going to do a power of good for those among us who need to be made whole tonight. And I feel that there is one among you who carries a burden in his belly which has been plaguing him for some time and that this burden needs to be loosed, in the name of JEEEESSSUUUUSSSS.'

That bastard Jeff, he'd set me up! Reverend Jim was obviously referring to me. I wasn't just being paranoid, was I?

'And I can feel that this burden can be lifted, if only you ask that it be done in the name of JEEEEESSSUUUUUSSSSS!'

There was that whooshing again. Yep, he was definitely talking about me, and now he was even *looking* at me. So was everyone else, for that matter – including Jeff, who was grinning widely.

'So come forth, brother, and be made whole . . . come forth and accept the Lord Jesus Christ as your personal Lord and Saviour,' he shouted.

I'd already tried that with Pastor Ray, with zilch result, but the pressure was on so I went forward and was immediately pounced on. Two of the band members grabbed my shoulders and Reverend Jim slapped a big clammy palm on my forehead and started chanting the biggest load of mumbo-jumbo I'd ever heard, occasionally finishing a passage off with another whooshing 'JEEESSSSUUUSSSSS'. The guys on my shoulders were trying to drag me onto the floor to demonstrate how powerful the healing was, but the floor didn't look that clean and I wasn't about to lie on it. The harder they dragged, the more I fought. They seemed to be getting pretty cheesed off with me, and when Reverend Jim eventually lifted his hand off my forehead and pronounced me healed, I had the unmitigated gall to say, 'Well actually, it feels like it's still there' – whereupon they started all over again, rather more roughly this time. They were becoming quite annoyed that I wasn't healed. I was making them look bad, I guess.

Then I had an epiphany. I could leave, right now. I had free will. I could just get the hell out of this nuthouse and make a run for it and never look back. I brushed them aside and made for the door.

'Don't go, brother! Don't go!' Reverend Jim shouted behind me. 'Don't turn your back on the Lord! Wide is the path to destruction and narrow the path to salvation. Come back and stride the narrow path with us, brother ... in JEEESSUUSSS' name.'

But I was out of there and into my car and tearing away before I remembered that Jeff had come with me and that I'd left him behind. But I wasn't going back. He could catch a bus home, couldn't he? Anyway, I was done with him and his holy-rolling buddies.

I was very cool with him when he came into my office the next day. 'You should have stayed,' he said. ' You really should have stayed.'

'Look, those guys were getting pretty scary, don't you think?' I said.

'Not as scary as the fires of hell,' he said.

'Well, how do they know there are fires there anyway?' I said. 'What sort of God barbecues His own creation?'

He wasn't hanging round to listen to that sort of talk, so he left me to my labours. I was pretty busy: there was an ad for a discount electrical warehouse that had to be turned into a 60-second spot by lunchtime. I glanced at one of the T S Eliot quotes on my desk – 'Do I dare . . . disturb the universe?' – took another swig of Mylanta and started typing.

A Mantra by Any Other Name

When the guy wearing the saffron-coloured turban appeared at the other end of the newsroom, I knew that whatever story he was involved with, it would somehow find its way to me. I was, after all, the local newspaper's resident weirdo correspondent.

After I arrived in Rockhampton, I had set the pace for what was to follow by doing a story about a Telecom technician who had been sacked for wearing a kaftan to work. I was assigned the job of wearing one at work just to see if that would actually interfere with a person's ability to do their job. I borrowed one from one of the women in the office and, I swear, that was the first and last time I ever wore one of her frocks. I donned the kaftan for a few hours and pottered around the office in it, much to the amusement of my workmates and the news editor, a bloke with a twisted sense of humour who had come up with the idea in the first place.

I wasn't silly enough to wear it out in the street, though, and I did all my work by phone that morning. It certainly didn't impede me around the office but it felt a bit weird hitching it up when I went to the men's room. I got the hem of the kaftan caught under one of the wheels of my ergonomic chair at one stage, but apart from that all was well. So I wrote an article about how easy it was to actually work in a kaftan. It appeared in the following day's newspaper accompanied by a picture of me, kaftan-clad, notebook at the ready. Kamahl would have understood where I was coming from but not everyone got it, and there were suggestions made in the daily letters page that I was, at the very least, effeminate, at worst a screaming queen. One correspondent, a bigot who was a well-known supporter of the Australian League of Rights — a right-wing Christian fundamentalist watchdog group — suggested that I was a hermaphrodite and an abomination in the eyes of God. I suggested an editor's reply pointing out that Jesus and the disciples wore kaftans too, but the boss passed on that.

This business marked me as the one who would be called on whenever something weird came up, or whenever someone weird came in, because even though I wore a business shirt and tie, I had long hair and John Lennon glasses so I was obviously a hippie. I glanced over again after a few minutes to see the tall slim bloke attached to the turban still sitting patiently in the small interviewing lounge just near the editor's glass fishbowl of an office. Everyone seemed to be ignoring the guy.

Mind you, had his gender been different, the youthful, testosterone-fuelled newsroom would have been a hive of activity, with the mostly young male reporters fighting over the prospect of an interview. There had been a rather unseemly episode the week before when an attractive young PR chick from the south had arrived in the office unannounced. That had everyone sitting up at their desks, sniffing the wind like those prairie dogs you see in *National Geographic* magazines. The woman had been ushered into the editor's office quicker than you could say 'male chauvinist pig' and there was a hell of a hubbub in the newsroom, everyone vying for the job of interviewing her, regardless of why she was in town. As it turned out, she had something to do with the Cattlemen's Union. When the editor – let's call him Old Jim – finally came out to talk to the turbaned one, several of my colleagues left the room.

'This one's got your name written all over it, Brownie,' said one as he absconded.

Meanwhile, down the end of the newsroom where the morning sun streamed in, I could see Old Jim scratching his head as the fellow explained himself. Now Jim wasn't exactly used to dealing with people in turbans. In the headgear department he favoured Akubras or the occasional pork-pie hat. Conservative to the core, he was convinced that his young reporters were dope-smoking communists bent on sedition – and to tell the truth, he wasn't entirely wrong on that score. His conservatism was tinged with eccentricity, though, which made it a bit more palatable. He liked to drink red wine at his desk in the evening and often succeeded in spilling half of it down his shirtfront. We used to pinch the occasional bottle from his stock after hours and he would go ballistic when he discovered one missing.

A Mantra by Any Other Name

The wine stains never quite came out of his shirts and with his general dishevelment and tousled hair he seemed quite mad at times. His image wasn't helped by the spectacles he was constantly pushing back up onto the bridge of his nose. He had done a home-made repair job on them and they were held together in the middle by a couple of band-aids which formed a distracting nodule in the middle of his face. It was a sort of absent-minded professor look.

On top of this, he was generally unable to remember our names, and referred to everyone as 'matey'. On this morning he had forgotten mine, again. 'That boy!' he shouted, pushing his spectacles up on his nose again and peering into the middle distance where I sat, alone. 'That boy with the hair!'

I closed the surfing magazine I had been reading inside the newspaper and sauntered over.

'This is . . . ' he said, pausing for a moment, scratching his head and looking vague.

'Dadaji,' the man offered gently. I shook hands with Dadaji and we sat down for a bit of a chat while Old Jim scuttled back into his office and shut the door. I opened my notebook and he began his spiel about being on a tour of Queensland to spread the good word about meditation and help people achieve inner peace.

'So where are you based?' I asked.

'In the Blue Mountains, but we are always travelling.'

'Have you been to Queensland before?' I asked.

'No, but some of my brothers have and they say the people here are very responsive.'

'As long as you're not wearing a kaftan,' I said. 'So what is actually the purpose of your visit?'

'I am part of a movement which simply aims to make the world a better place,' he said. 'By teaching people to look inwards rather than outwards, a revolution is possible... but a peaceful revolution of course. We aim to spread the message that through yoga, meditation and God-consciousness world peace will finally be possible.'

'Well, we could sure use some inner peace in old Rock Vegas,' I said. I was thinking of a fight I'd witnessed the night before at the Casa Del Quay, a nightclub just down the road from the newspaper. It was one of our field offices.

'Indeed,' said Dadaji, with the hint of an Indian accent. 'It is needed everywhere most urgently.' He didn't really look Indian but I guess he had spent time there. His name was probably Daryl Smith or something equally prosaic, but you probably wouldn't expect someone by that name to be carrying the torch for spiritual enlightenment. And how many Daryls have you met who wear turbans? Dadaji's origins seemed ambiguous, which might all have been part of the act. The mild Indian accent, the wispy beard (my old man would have called it 'bum fluff'), the turban and the subcontinental outfit – it looked kind of Punjabi – couldn't hide the fact that the guy was obviously not Indian, despite the exotic persona he was projecting.

'So what can we do for you?' I asked.

'Perhaps we can have a story in the newspaper about our talks and meditation training here in Rockhampton. Yes?' He wobbled his head the way Indians do.

'Yes, well I'm sure we can do a little story.' So we chatted about yoga and meditation and he spruiked their supposed health and social benefits. I couldn't quite get a handle on which religion he belonged to.

But it was a very slow news day. It often was early in the week in Rocky: the really exciting things usually happened towards the weekend, when people had drunk more. So we needed bumph to fill the paper, and it didn't really matter whether he was a nutter or the reincarnation of the Buddha.

'Are you interested in spiritual matters yourself?' Dadaji asked.

'As a matter of fact I am,' I said. 'I'm a bit confused about it all but I'm certainly interested.'

My conversion to Catholicism just a couple of years earlier somehow hadn't stopped my spiritual searching – although I'd learnt that wasn't something one went on about too much in the newsroom. I didn't confine myself to Catholic worship, though, by any means, and since arriving in Rockhampton I had been attending Catholic and Anglican services, which was handy for a reporter because both denominations thought I was with them. By working both sides of the street I had most of the town covered. I was even invited to the Anglican bishop's residence on the strength of my churchgoing and never had the heart to dispel the myth that I was a committed Anglican.

But I found it difficult to confine myself to mainstream Christianity, and was also open to Oriental spirituality, probably a legacy of growing up in Hong Kong surrounded by Taoists and Buddhists – not to mention capitalists. My bedside table was groaning with books that had an Eastern bent – stuff by Bede Griffiths, Alan Watts, D T Suzuki – and I had been dabbling in meditation techniques for years with little success. Whenever I would try to sit quietly and fill my mind with peaceful nothingness, terrible intrusive thoughts and visions would interrupt – nuclear holocausts, bikini girls, and flashbacks to episodes of *Gilligan's Island*. I had been to some meditation evenings at an ashram (it was just a house with no furniture in it, really) back home on the Gold Coast but found the practice gave me a headache and little else. I hadn't given up, though.

Zen meditation, which I'd been having a crack at teaching myself recently, in secret, seemed particularly difficult and required sitting very uncomfortably with knees folded underneath on a hard floor. When Zen novices are having trouble with this and nod off, or don't hold the right position correctly, their masters apparently give them a bit of a touch-up with a length of bamboo. The way my technique was going, a piece of four-by-two with a four-inch nail sticking out of it would have been more appropriate. At home in a sleepy Rockhampton suburb, I had spent hours trying to master this meditation technique but got nothing for my troubles other than dents in my knees from the seagrass matting, which I once accidentally set on fire with the candle I was using to concentrate my thoughts. Foolishly, perhaps, I talked about some of this during my interview with Dadaji and he nodded sagely.

'One can't just pick up meditation, like a cold, one needs

to be taught true meditation,' he said, with that fake Indian lilt. 'One needs a teacher. And when the student is ready, the teacher usually appears.'

'I'm afraid I might be a bit of a lost cause in the meditation stakes,' I said, realising he had delivered a veiled offer to teach me how to meditate.

'Being lost is the first step towards being found and of stepping onto the beginning of your true path,' he said. I was tempted to ask whether he might like me to try snatching the pebble from his hand at this stage, but fought off the urge.

Later I tapped out a little story about how the good folk of Rocky could expand their consciousness for next to no capital outlay by attending Dadaji's yoga and meditation sessions, and at the end of the day's work did what I always did — adjourned to the Criterion Hotel next door to the newspaper's offices on historic Quay Street for some libations with the other reporters. When not attending church services, trying to meditate, reading books on Eastern religion or writing poetry, I spent a lot of time in Rockhampton drinking, which seemed, in those days, to be *de rigueur* for any young journo. I took Jack Kerouac, Ernest Hemingway and other literary lushes as my models — which didn't really dovetail with my metaphysical leanings. Hard to meditate when you're pissed.

I was, however, interested enough to intend going to Dadaji's public talk and meditation lesson. His style sounded easier than the Zen version, after all, and might save my knees. I did have a free night too, but then the work roster was changed and I was stuck on the two-till-10 shift that day, a long haul that consisted mainly of police rounds. That shift had been fertile ground for me as far as reporting experience went, and had already won me an award – the only one I have ever received in journalism – for Story of the Year when I lucked onto a mass food-poisoning at a pensioner's dinner. There were no fatalities, luckily, although I got the feeling some of my colleagues wished there had been. A mass food-poisoning is always good news – for the news desk that is, not the victims. A few years later, when Bhagwan Shree Rajneesh's right-hand woman, Ma Sheela, tried to poison some recalcitrant locals in Oregon, I couldn't help thinking back to Rocky and my moment of front-page glory. But such stories were few and far between, and night work mostly consisted of working the phones and going on take-away Chinese food runs for the sub-editors. The chief sub-editor was a jolly enough fellow, for a sadist, and delighted in getting me to rewrite story intros anything up to a dozen times. So that kept me busy, too.

On the night that I had planned to attend the meditation workshop I was in the office ringing around the region's police stations, fishing for bad news instead. Of course, when you go looking for bad news you can usually find some, and after a half-dozen calls I got a bite from a rather weary constable.

'There's been a nasty smash on the Marlborough stretch,' he yawned. 'The Sarge is out now attending it.'

'Anyone hurt?' I asked.

'Oh, mate, I don't know yet,' he said. I turned, put my

hand over the mouthpiece and shouted across to the sub-editors' desk. 'There's been a bingle on the Marlborough stretch if you're interested!'

'Was it fatal?' asked the chief sub.

'I'm just trying to find out,' I said. He looked excited at the possibility. I went back to the constable.

'Actually the Sarge is coming in now... hang on,' he said.

'Can you ask him if there were any fatalities?'

'Hold your horses, buddy,' he said as they conferred in the background. Then he confirmed that there were none – just minor injuries – and I relayed that to the subs' desk.

'Damn it,' the chief sub said.

The next day I was on the late shift again so I went into town in the morning to have coffee and do some browsing in a bookstore, where I ran into Dadaji. The turban poking above a book stand was a dead giveaway. He greeted me like a long-lost pal.

'Sorry I didn't get to your talk last night,' I said.

'Oh, never mind... it went very well,' he said. 'The hall was three-quarters full.'

'So there's some life in the old town after all. When are you leaving?'

'Oh, I have a few more days here yet and I think we should get together before I leave,' he said. 'If you're still interested in learning something about meditation, that is?'

'Well, yes, I guess I am. As I mentioned, I haven't had much success so far, but maybe that can be turned around with a little expert tuition.'

'I am staying with some people up on the hills and meeting with people there in the evenings,' he said. 'Are you free Friday night?'

What did I usually do Friday nights? Watch telly with my housemates, drinking red wine until we couldn't sit up straight in our chairs any more. Or we'd smoke some more of the horrendous weed that a friend had been passing around. Dadaji scribbled down the address for me in a small notepad. 'Will you come at 8 p.m?'

'Gosh, I don't know. There's so much happening here in Rocky I can't imagine where I'd find the time,' I said. He looked at me, obviously confused. 'Only joking,' I assured him. 'I'll be there.'

When I saw the name and address I recognised it immediately as belonging to a well-to-do couple, by Rocky standards – she had a dress shop, he was a solicitor. I had been to a party there some months earlier as part of a rent-a-crowd of fashionable young folk – they being in their late thirties, which seemed moribund to my friends and me. My recollection was a bit vague but it was up in the Berserker Range just north of town, and it had been a dope-laden affair. Between the evening fog and the internal haze at that party, it was all a bit of a blur now. But it seemed typical of them to pick up a wandering ascetic like Dadaji – a sort of poor man's Maharishi.

Come Friday evening I knocked off, went home, had some grilled cheese on toast, showered and got ready for my meditation lesson. Does one wear aftershave to a meditation lesson? I asked myself as I looked in the mirror while cleaning my teeth. Well, probably not, but the fact of the matter was that the last time I was at the house on the hill it had been crawling with young women so I splashed on a few dollops of Brut 33 just in case. Yep, I had class.

'If anyone lights a match near you tonight you'll go up like a bloody bonfire,' said one of my housemates. 'You smell like a shearer on a Saturday night.'

'It's *Friday* night and, actually, I'm on my way to learn meditation,' I said. 'You just sit there and drink yourself into a stupor if it makes you feel better. But don't go riding that bloody pushbike again tonight, okay? Not while there's nobody around to pick you up.' He occasionally took to his racing bike when stoned or tanked and usually came back with grazes all over.

I left him in his cups and drove through North Rockhampton, which was as dead as a doornail even on a Friday night, and up the winding road to the mountain eyrie owned by . . . now what the hell were their names?

When the lady of the house opened the door I just said: 'Well, hello again!'

'Hi, Phil,' she said, remembering me but sensing that I had forgotten her name. 'It's Grace.'

She was wearing a prayer shirt with no bra underneath. It took a Herculean effort to keep looking her in the eye.

'You're here to see Dadaji of course,' Grace said. 'Isn't he marvellous? I have already done my session with him and got my secret mantra.'

'Secret mantra?' I said, intrigued. 'I didn't know there were secret mantras involved.'

'Oh yes,' Grace said, leading me inside. 'You need a secret mantra to access your inner core. It's sort of like a password to your soul.'

'Really?' I said, fixing her with a very serious look. 'So what's yours?'

'But of course if I told you that it wouldn't be secret any more, would it?'

What brilliant logic.

In the lounge room, where Grace had led me, there were maybe a dozen people sitting around in various stages of semi-consciousness. A few, including one girl I knew, seemed to be as high as kites, and the familiar smell of marijuana pervaded the room, barely covered up by the incense that was burning in several portals. Dadaji seemed to be the only one who was even vaguely alert, and he looked relieved when I arrived, apparently happy to be given an excuse to remove himself from the stoned lounge-room crowd. I had recognised a couple of other people by now, including two guys from a new wave band called the Grinders which I had written a story about a few weeks earlier. By day they toiled at the meatworks, by night they thrashed out punk music at various seedy pubs. They made feeble gestures of recognition and continued nodding their heads to the music — Pink Floyd's *Dark Side of the Moon*.

'They are very nice people,' Dadaji said. 'But all that drug smoking is not helpful for God-consciousness. Not at all. Now come, follow me.'

He led me into a room, which was obviously the man of the house's study (was his name Paul?). One wall was a full-length window with a wonderful view out across the mountains and down over a flat expanse to the coast. Lights twinkled far below but were quickly extinguished when Dadaji pulled a curtain across the view. So this was the moment of truth? I was about to learn to meditate properly at last – no more sore knees and wayward thoughts, no more domestic fires, no more wasted hours – this was the real deal.

'We don't want any distractions,' Dadaji said as he sat on the floor and assumed the lotus position. 'Please, won't you join me?'

'Um, sure,' I said, sitting down and attempting to emulate his position, which wasn't easy. 'But I'm not very supple I'm afraid. I'm not sure if I can sit like this for too long.'

'It is fine,' he said. 'Just sit and you will become comfortable.' Dadaji stroked his wispy beard for a minute and then looked at me.

'We shall talk a little first,' he said. 'Tell me something about what you believe. For example, do you think there is a meaning to life?'

'Well, either there is, or there isn't,' I said.

'But you go to church and have studied religion,' he said. 'Does this not indicate that you believe life has a meaning and that you are seeking it?'

'I may be seeking it but it's bloody elusive,' I said. 'And as for meaning, well, I guess I look at it this way – Jesus and Buddha make a lot of sense to me, on the one hand, but on the other, the whole business of life can seem like a rather black joke at times.'

'A joke?' he said, his head wobbling a little in the Indian fashion, even though he was as Australian as I was. 'Oh, surely not a joke?'

'Well, not a very funny one,' I said. 'I mean, existence all seems rather cruel sometimes – being born into this vulnerable human form with the consciousness that we have, only to be snuffed out in the end just as we're getting the hang of it. It seems bloody cruel really – that we exist as sentient beings, with all the knowledge of our existence, our frailty and our finiteness, knowing all the while that we are doomed to extinction. I mean, what's that all about?'

I was impressed with my own summation but he shook his head. 'But you don't believe things are that bleak, surely?'

'Every other day I do,' I said. 'Today's my alternate day, though, and I'm feeling that the universe is filthy with meaning tonight.'

'Ah,' he said, going all subcontinental again. 'It is your sense of humour.' He became quiet then, looked down and closed his eyes. I sensed that I should do the same but then he opened his eyes again.

'Before we meditate and you receive your mantra you must purify yourself,' he said.

'Oh yes,' I said. 'And how do I do that?'

'With ritual washing of your extremities, so you are cleansed in body before becoming cleansed in mind.'

'Riiiiighht,' I said. All of a sudden I had this horrific vision of Dadaji and me sitting in a bath together, him sponging my back. I fought back the suspicion that this was all a ruse and that he was actually just keen on me.

'Beyond that door,' he pointed to a closed door opposite the one we came in through, 'is the bathroom. Please wash your face, your hands, your feet and your private parts, and after that we can begin.'

Warning bells started going off in my head and all of a sudden I thought I felt a panic attack coming on. 'Is that really necessary?' I asked. 'I mean, I showered before I came.'

'It is a normal part of your preparation,' he insisted.

'Cleanliness is next to godliness, I guess,' I said as I got up a bit gingerly, unfolding myself from the human pretzel I had become trying to achieve the lotus position. This washing thing seemed a bit rich, but then I was always a stickler for detail, so I was determined to go through with it – even if that meant doing something that seemed tantamount to onanism.

The bathroom was spacious but a bit dim even after I turned a light on. The bulb must have been of a very low wattage, I figured, as I washed my hands and splashed my face. There was a washer on the side of the basin, which I used for my feet, and then it came to the interesting bit. I could just say I had done it, I thought, and skip the nether region, but then I might not be able to keep a straight face. I really did want to learn to meditate – and wouldn't having a secret mantra help me immeasurably in life? I couldn't be sure about that but hell, I'd come this far. So I dropped my trousers and dipped my wedding tackle in the basin with the idea of having a very cursory splash. Of course I felt quite ridiculous.

And just as I did that, the other door to the bathroom opened and there was a glaring light. I had obviously turned on a minor light, and whoever had just come in had found the main one and switched it on to find me in, well, what would in normal circumstances be seen as a compromising position. When I looked up I saw that it was Grace's husband, who was looking a bit dishevelled and quite shocked.

'What the bloody hell do you think you're playing at?' he asked. 'And who the bloody hell are you anyway!?'

I wasn't sure which question to answer first. 'Um, look, I can explain this easily,' I said.

'Listen, mate, if you want to have a wank, do it in the privacy of your own home and not in my bathroom,' he said, and then he fixed me with a stare. 'Aren't you that guy from the paper?'

'Well, yes, I am,' I said, tucking myself in and pulling up my trousers. I half put my hand out in greeting before thinking better of it.

'Look, I'm here to see Dadaji and this is all just part of his meditation ritual. I know it seems ridiculous but he insisted that I had to do this before we meditate. It's part of a purification ritual. You've been through this yourself, haven't you?'

'No bloody way. I told my missus that I wasn't having anything to do with that Indian dole bludger,' he said.

'Ah, I don't think he's actually Indian,' I said, but he wasn't listening.

He turned and started shouting, 'Grace, Grace . . . for Christ's sake, when are you going to clear these hippie poofs out of here so I can get some sleep!' He went out, slamming the door. Grace came in then, apologised profusely and insisted I go back to Dadaji to finish my meditation lesson.

'I'm so sorry about Paul,' she said. 'Terribly upsetting when you're trying to meditate. Bit of a misunderstanding, that's all. We'll leave you to it now.'

I was mortified at being sprung with my pants down, and totally flustered. I went back to the room where Dadaji sat, not exactly in the mood for any contemplation. Dadaji had obviously heard the ruckus but was either oblivious to such things or just pretending to be, to prove his credentials as a swami.

'Misunderstandings abound,' he said. 'But we cannot let the universal mind be disturbed by such ripples in the pond of consciousness. Now let us meditate.'

He closed his eyes and I closed mine. I tried to calm down as he started a spiel about peace and tranquillity . . . something to do with merging with the Godhead. He spoke in a sort of lulling monotone, the Indian accent waxing and waning as he went. Then there was a bit of chanting and then some low unintelligible ranting, then some quiet time. I was a bit rattled but tried hard to concentrate . . . picturing the cosmos and attempting to become one with it but generally failing to do so. My mind strayed awfully and I found myself thinking about everything from sex to my bank account to what I would be doing that weekend. But my thoughts particularly kept coming back to the look of disgust on Paul's face when he'd found me with my crown jewels in his bathroom basin.

Eventually Dadaji cut in on my frantic thought patterns. 'It is time to receive your secret mantra,' he said, rubbing his hands together and then placing them palm-down on his knees.

'Um, okayyyy,' I said, trying to sound grateful as he leant forward and whispered something in my ear. I was finding it hard to concentrate and had really lost my meditating momentum.

'I'm sorry, I didn't quite catch that,' I said as his lips brushed my ear.

He leant towards me again. 'Baba,' he whispered and then repeated, 'Baba.'

'Baba?' I said. 'As in black sheep? That's it?' I didn't mean to sound disappointed.

'Yes, that is it,' he said. 'Keep it close to your heart and never utter it except in the depths of your meditation. When you meditate, repeating your mantra aloud at first and then silently within, it will connect you with the Godhead and can lead to great spiritual progress. So, begin.'

'Sure.' I closed my eyes again and spent a bit of time muttering 'Baba, baba, baba' out loud, and then just thinking the word to myself as we sat there in silence for a few minutes. It all seemed too easy. We went on like that for about half an hour or so and then, suddenly, it seemed the session was over. We both untangled ourselves and got up. My foot had gone to sleep so I had to do a bit of a surfie stomp to get it back to normal again. Then we went back out to the living room, which was a bit depleted now with only a trickle of guests left lounging around.

A Mantra by Any Other Name

'We're leaving,' said one of the girls as we came in. 'Paul's being a real arsehole. Can't handle his piss, or his dope, for that matter.'

'Paul is very tired,' Grace said diplomatically, adding to me, 'I'm sorry about before.'

'Not at all,' I said, looking at my watch, embarrassed. 'And actually I have to go now myself.' I said my goodbyes and promised Dadaji that I would meditate and use my secret mantra well in the coming weeks.

'I may not be back again for a while but one of my brothers will be coming up here in a few months, so I'll ask him to come and see you,' he smiled. 'He can check your progress.'

'Sure, sure, tell him to look me up,' I said, keen to get out of the joint before I ran into Paul again.

Later, I lay in bed wondering if the universe was eternal, who had created eternity, and what I would have for breakfast. As I lay there I decided to try out my secret mantra. I concentrated and thought 'Baba, baba, baba, baba' for a while but it didn't seem to have any obvious effect. Over the next few weeks I spent several hours sitting in great discomfort on my bedroom floor meditating myself into a stupor chanting 'Baba'. I got sore knees but little else, and figured that I might have needed a few follow-up lessons to get the hang of this meditating business. Being a worrier, I really wanted to get into a state where thought was banished and day-to-day problems expunged from the mind, but it never happened. I felt guilty that I got more inner peace watching television. I was obviously an utter failure as a meditator, and was reminded of that several months later when I looked up from my desk and saw another bloke wearing a saffron turban sitting in the waiting area at the end of the newsroom.

'Another one of your mates,' my colleague said.

'I don't think so,' I said. 'If anyone is looking for me, I'm not here.' I went to the men's room, locked myself in a cubicle and waited there for a quarter of an hour or so. When I came back, the man had gone. I sat down at my desk and found a small, white envelope tucked into my typewriter keyboard.

'The bloke with the orange tea towel on his head left that for you,' my colleague said.

'I hope there's money in it,' I said. I tore it open and took out a small slip of paper, which was folded in half. I opened it and there was one word written on it in pencil . . . 'Baba'.

On the Other Side of the Couch

'You seem a little depressed,' said Dr Bernini, patting his head. There wasn't a hair out of place.

'Maybe I am,' I said.

'Does that worry you?'

'I couldn't care less,' I said.

'Aahhh,' he said.

'Is that significant?' I asked.

'It might be.'

Could the guy be a bit more specific?

He got up, walked across the immaculate room to where a small mirror hung on the wall, and examined himself in it. He adjusted his tie and brushed some lint off his lapels. Dr Bernini was, I figured, the best-dressed man in Surfers Paradise. Every other middle-aged bloke in town was wandering around in a safari suit or shorts and long socks but he looked like an Armani ad. His demeanour was as cool as his clothing and he spoke in a measured way, as if keen not to ruffle himself. As for his skill as a psychiatrist, well, I wasn't at all sure about that. He came back and sat down, oblivious to my bemused look.

'Depression is caused by an imbalance of certain chemicals in the brain.' He tapped his skull in case I wasn't sure where mine was. 'We now have drugs which can fix that, luckily. In fact, I'll prescribe you a course of antidepressants, and you will be through this in no time.' He passed me an information sheet about depression and medication and asked me a few more cursory questions, but I could sense that his heart wasn't really in it. I got the impression that he actually wanted me out of there as soon as possible. By the way he kept looking at his watch, I guessed he might have a lunch date. This was annoying really because I'd been kind of looking forward to some deep Freudian analysis.

My dad had died the year before and I was pretty emotionally messed up, and I figured that qualified me for some serious couch time. I mean, Woody Allen spent several decades in psychoanalysis, which seems a bit steep. But I must warrant at least a few months . . .

Maybe it was just that Dr Bernini didn't want his couch messed up by people lolling all over it. It was spotless and appeared to be brand new. I looked longingly at it but he just wrote me a prescription and told me to make an appointment for a month's time. A month? Would I last that long?

In the meantime I had the prescription filled and started taking the yippee beans. He promised they'd have an almost immediate effect, and they certainly did because within a week I was a virtual zombie. I'd wake up in the morning, dry-mouthed, hardly able to remember my own name, and would drag my carcass through the days like the living dead. The last time a prescription drug had any such effect on me was in my senior year at school, when a GP at Broadbeach had prescribed Mogadon because I was experiencing some anxiety. Who doesn't in Grade 12? I remember the consultation vividly because he'd seemed convinced that my anxiety had something to do with my love life.

'Are you in love?' he'd asked.

'No.'

'Not at all?'

'Not at all.'

'Because love can be difficult.'

'I am certainly not in love,' I'd said.

I'm thinking he might have actually suspected I was in love with a boy, but who knows? Anyway, he seemed disappointed somehow that I wasn't lovelorn for either gender and quickly ejected me with a script for Mogadon. I took a tablet that evening and soon found myself sliding along the walls as I went down the hallway of the upstairs part of our house, where our parents had so wisely corralled their three children. And now, with these anti-depressants, I was shuffling around like a geriatric in need of a walking frame. I wasn't keen on such zombiehood again. Prescription drugs and I didn't seem to get on.

I went back to our family GP, a well-known hypochondriac whom my father always used to greet with: 'Gee, you're not looking too well today.' I complained to him about Dr Bernini's diffidence and the extreme effect of the pills.

'I'm taking them,' I said. 'But now I don't know whether I'm Arthur or Martha.'

'Well, I could refer you to someone else,' he said checking his own pulse as he spoke.

He reached into his drawer, pulled out some silver foil, extracted a tablet and swigged it down with a little paper cup full of water. 'There's a new psychiatrist who has just moved here from England. He's supposed to be very good. Would you like to try him?'

Jesus, here I was in my mid-twenties and I was already shrink-shopping! I said I would, happily, and within a week I was sitting in the waiting room of a certain Dr Roger Reeve. He soon appeared, gently ushering the previous patient out before ushering me in.

'Nice couch,' I said, plonking myself down on it.

'You can use the couch but feel free to sit in the chair if you'd prefer.'

'Don't you guys ever use the couch nowadays?'

'I think you've been watching too many movies,' he smiled. 'I do use it very occasionally but I find people tend to fall asleep. It could be something to do with the sound of my voice, of course.' The man had a sense of humour, which seemed a good sign. 'Besides,' he went on, 'I like to work on what I call "the other side of the couch", which I suppose is my way of saying I like to work a little differently. I find if people start on the couch, they never quite get off it – literally and metaphorically. The couch is very comfortable, and in a sense many people don't really want to get off it because they don't want to change. In the same way, some hang on to their illness because it's comfortable – the known rather than the unknown. But of course on the other side of the couch there is an entire world of wellness and a scary world of personal responsibility.'

I nodded. 'I'll sit then,' I said, moving to a comfy chair half-facing him. I was already feeling vastly more at ease than I had with Dr Bernini, who seemed to have turned anal retention into an art form. Dr Reeve was immediately more approachable and a lot more relaxed. He was dressed well too, but there was just a hint of dishevelment about him and he had a small goatee beard. He reminded me of the dotty British comedian Michael Bentine, one of the original Goons, if your memory goes back that far. He had a large, rose-gold wedding ring on one hand and a signet ring bearing a cross insignia on his other hand; he looked like he could have been a candidate for Archbishop of Canterbury. Hopefully he wasn't going to ask me to kiss his ring. I did notice some religious books in the shelves behind him too, as well as the thick psychiatric tomes.

'Are you interested in theology?' I asked, since I was.

'Yes, I am,' he said.

'You're a churchgoer?'

'Anglican by preference but philosophically ecumenical. And you?'

'A very confused Catholic convert.'

'Good Lord, I didn't think there was such a thing any more.'

I filled him in on my situation and how unhappy I was taking Dr Bernini's pills.

'They can help but they can also hinder,' Dr Reeve confessed. 'You may well have a chemical basis to your depression but there are other factors involved, are there not? I mean, you've mentioned that your father died only very recently, yes?'

'That's right,' I said.

'Well, if you weren't depressed after that, you'd be a psychopath.'

I nodded. I wasn't a psychopath? This was good news.

'We all go through these dark nights of the soul at times, and sometimes medication is helpful in these matters. But sometimes I feel it's better to actually experience the grief, or whatever feeling you're feeling, and move through it. The only way out is through . . . I'm not sure who said that. Sounds like a pop song, don't you think?'

This session was going swimmingly compared to my visit to Dr Bernini, who had said little and was keen to get me out of his office as soon as he could and to pump me full of drugs to keep me quiet. Dr Reeve, meanwhile, was chatty as hell — and in fact seemed to be doing more talking than me. I felt like I was having an audience with a well-read country parson rather than a psychiatrist. Mind you, he seemed as out of place in Tinsel Town as Dr Bernini. His office was a bookish den, curtains partly drawn to take the edge off the light, but through the gap in them I could see outside — another perfect day in Surfers Paradise, with the skyscrapers towering away in the distance.

'How the heck did you end up on the Gold Coast?' I asked.

'Well, I came to do a locum for another doctor about a year ago and we decided we'd stay,' he said. 'There's certainly no lack of business opportunity here for someone in my field. I mean, it's nice and glossy on the surface, but there are problems. A lot of people seem to move here to escape themselves but are a little surprised to find they've brought their problems with them.'

'But this is the fabulous Gold Coast,' I protested. 'Nothing bad ever happens here. It's all sun and surf . . . '

'. . . and dysfunction,' he said, completing my sentence. 'Never mind. It'll keep me busy for years.' The irreverence was a bit of a surprise but refreshing. Meanwhile, he suggested I cut back on my dosage of the dreaded tablets and come back to see him a week later, which I did. And the week after that.

The sessions with Dr Reeve were helpful but I was still in what they used to call 'a blue funk'. I was pretty dark with life in general and had developed a fairly doom-laden world view. I mean, one is not a very happy chappie if, when standing on a street corner waiting to cross the road, one has visions of the entire streetscape being vaporised by a hydrogen bomb. Such apocalyptic delusions pervaded my waking hours, and prophets of doom were magnets to me. Around this time there was a spectacular alignment of the planets called 'the Jupiter Effect', which, as far as I can recall, consisted of all the planets lining up on one side of the sun – an apparently rare event. Some New Age nuts and Bible prophecy loonies had earmarked this as ushering in the end of the world, and the date in question was only months away. I became convinced that the end may be nigh, and told Dr Reeve.

'Utter rot,' was his view. 'Piffle. I can't understand why so many people are so keen for the end to arrive. The evangelicals seem to be willing it on and as for these astrological nutters... it really doesn't bear thinking about. Unless you're depressed I suppose, in which case it would make perfect sense.'

'I suppose you're right,' I said.

'Even if they were right, there's nothing we could do about it, is there?'

'I suppose not.'

'We might as well make the most of things regardless. It's all in Ecclesiastes, isn't it?'

That didn't make me feel that much better, actually. I was in a downward spiral and was worrying 25 hours a day, and seemed to have lost my appetite completely. I was still taking the tablets, though on a lesser dose and getting nowhere. I was already thin but was also losing weight.

'I think we might give you a rest in hospital,' Dr Reeve said at our next session.

'Hospital!' I said. 'My old man said if you were ever sick, hospital was the last place you should go.'

'You're suffering from nervous exhaustion and, quite frankly, I think a rest in hospital for a few days will help.'

I was admitted to Pindara Private Hospital that afternoon. And it wasn't too bad in there at all. I had a television and a private room and hot and cold running nurses, plus three square meals a day, with morning and afternoon tea. I had my books with me and some pads to scrawl poems on should any happen to surface in between soap operas. It was great, actually, even if there wasn't anything actually wrong with me.

Lying back between the crisp new sheets in my hospital bed, I felt like Frederic Henry in *A Farewell to Arms* (I was attracted to Hemingway at the time – another depressive) though I hadn't exactly suffered anything like the horrors of the trenches. In fact we had absolutely nothing in common, though I did have a vague hope that, as in the novel, one of the more attractive nurses might take a shine to me. But they all seemed far too busy attending to the sick folk. Talk about selfish!

My mum came in to see me every day and brought me some fruitcake. She was worried, as usual, but seemingly glad I was under medical supervision. And Dr Reeve came in on his rounds every day. He was very jolly about it all even though I was, despite the escapism, mildly embarrassed to be there.

'Resting comfortably, as they say in the classics?'

'I feel like I'm in a scene from *Carry on Doctor*,' I said.

'I know what you mean,' he laughed. 'But it's awfully comfortable in here. I wouldn't mind a few days in this place myself.'

'Yes, well, you'll have to get your own room,' I said. 'But it is pretty swish. I feel like I've checked into a five-star hotel for the week and just haven't left my room.'

'It's wonderful, except for all the sick people,' he laughed.

'Yes, that's an inconvenience,' I said. 'If they could just clear them all out of here it would be much more agreeable.'

He sat down in a chair beside the bed and regarded the small pile of books on my bedside table. '*The Bell Jar, Death and Eternal Life, The Snows of Kilimanjaro and Other Stories* . . . not exactly what I call light reading!'

'No, I guess not,' I said. I had been sitting up in bed reading *Death and Eternal Life* by John Hick the day before when a friend and his girlfriend came in to visit. My mate had rung me later to say his girlfriend had asked him if I was dying.

'"No, he's not dying", I told her,' he'd said. '"He's just having a bit of a lie down."' I told Dr Reeve that and he was amused.

'My dear boy, we're all dying by degrees,' he said. 'The trick is to actually live before one does snuff it. After all, you only get one shot at it. This is not a dress rehearsal.'

This was of course quite a long time ago, but by some miracle he seemed to be channelling Dr Phil!

After five days in the sick-house the good doctor decided I was fit to rejoin the human race. I came out heavier than when I went in thanks to the hospital stodge I had stuffed myself with. I went back to see Dr Reeve the following week.

'You're looking rested,' he said.

'I guess so,' I said. 'But everything still seems a bit grey to me.'

'Grey is okay,' he said. 'Sometimes grey is the best we can hope for. Anyway, grey is better than black.'

And at the time that actually made sense to me.

Nil by Mouth

'You're nuts,' my cousin Peter said as we sped across the Sydney Harbour Bridge. 'Why do you need to go to a health farm anyway? You're built like a bloody whippet.'

'It's not a fat farm,' I explained. 'I don't want to lose weight. I want to purify my body.'

'I'm the one who should be going to a health farm,' he said. 'I actually need to be on a diet. Anyway, just remember, you know where I am if you decide you want to get the hell out of the place.'

Peter just couldn't get his head around the idea because he lived on cigarettes, beer and Chinese food. His idea of a health kick was forgoing barbecued pork buns for a day, so when I had explained to him that I expected to spend part of my two weeks' holiday from work at the Elysian Sanitarium fasting, he shook his head, uncomprehending.

'If you don't eat you don't shit, and if you don't shit you die,' he said, lighting a cigarette. 'Now are you sure you don't want to stop at Chatswood for a quick yum cha? A condemned man deserves a last meal.'

I shook my head. I just wanted to get to the place now and see what I'd let myself in for. I'd paid a hefty fee for the exercise, which, I hoped, would set me on the road to beaming health and spiritual enlightenment. I'd been reading all sorts of alternative health books in the preceding months and was convinced that since the body was the temple of the soul, it was time I cleaned up my act. There was a movement around at the time called Breatharianism, and Breatharians reckoned they could basically live on air alone, according to one of the wackier tomes I had consulted. There were various reports out of India of people living for years without food. They claimed that sunlight, air or *prana* (Sanskrit for breath) were sufficient to sustain life. I had read of an Indian ascetic, Prahladbhai Jani, who lived in a cave and claimed not to have eaten for 68 years. I didn't want to go that far but I'd got it in my head that a bodily cleansing would help me because, to tell the truth, I felt physically and mentally run down. I mean, I shouldn't have at the age of 26, but there you have it.

A friend who was a health nut and into this sort of thing had known someone who had apparently been to this sanitarium and came back raving about the experience. Impetuous as I was back then, I rang them up and booked myself in.

My colleagues thought I was nuts but that was nothing new. I took a couple of weeks' holiday from my job as a reporter on *The Gold Coast Bulletin* and flew to Sydney.

'So what do you know about the people who run this joint, anyway?' asked Peter as we began to put the suburban sprawl of Sydney behind us.

'Not very much at all,' I said, enjoying the scenery – stone cottages and green paddocks that made it look more like Ireland than the outskirts of Sin City.

'Probably some sort of cult,' he muttered. 'Anyway, like I said, you know where I am if you need me.'

We were in the vicinity of the sanitarium by now. I read out the directions I'd been given – the last landmark was a small corner store at a country crossroads. The Elysian Sanitarium was about 2 kms past that. A discreet sign above a small letterbox announced the location, finally, and we bumped down a shady driveway and pulled up out the front of a small group of bungalow-like buildings. I hauled my bag out of the boot.

'Do you want me to come in with you?' Peter asked.

'What are you, my boyfriend? I'll be fine.'

'It's bloody quiet around here,' he said. 'Creepy.'

'Mate, it's a bloody health centre, not Club Med,' I said. 'I'll be alright, don't worry. Thanks for the lift.'

I waved him off and looked around. He was right, it was a bit creepy, and to add to that creepiness a gaunt, bearded face suddenly appeared at one of the windows, staring out at me. It was the sort of face you'd expect to see staring from behind the cell bars of solitary confinement on Devil's Island, I thought, as the curtain was quickly pulled closed again. Before I had time to wonder whether I'd made a big mistake coming here, the front door opened and a rather chubby, jolly, swarthy woman burst out the door and came towards me.

'Welcome to Elysian!' she bellowed and pumped my hand. I couldn't help noticing a hint of five o'clock shadow on her upper lip.

'Hello, Brown's the name,' I said enthusiastically.

'Yes, yes, of course it is!' she said. 'Come in, we've been expecting you. We'll fix you up in no time. Or rather, we'll help you fix yourself. It's amazing what healing powers the body really has... if we can just unlock them. I'm Mrs Goldman... come in, come in and meet Dr Goldman. He'll give you your examination before we show you to your room.'

'Examination?'

'Oh, yes, yes, definitely,' she said. 'He's very thorough. Have to make sure you're up to it.'

I wondered how 'up to it' I was supposed to be. I mean, one of the reasons I was here was because I didn't really feel 'up to it'. Mrs Goldman led me past the reception area, knocked on a large wooden door and took me into the doctor's rooms. I felt the joint must be kosher with doctors in charge.

'Just wait here, he'll be in shortly,' she said.

The doctor arrived moments later, and the first thing I noticed was that he too was a bit paunchy. I guess I had expected some obscenely vital, silver-haired specimen glowing with rude health. He was actually a bit pasty-faced too, and his thick hair looked positively greasy.

'Ah, Mr Brown,' he said, coming towards me with a fat outstretched hand. He gave me one of those invertebrate handshakes, limp and doughy. 'Good, good, now let's strip down to our underpants shall we, and we'll see what's what.'

Presumably he meant just me. So I sat on the edge of his examining bench while he pressed and prodded, listened to my heart, took my blood pressure and then proceeded to weigh me. His hands were freezing as well as flaccid.

'Well, nothing too serious,' he declared after jotting a few things down. 'But you certainly could use a little bit of what we have to offer.'

'Yes,' I agreed.

'Peace and quiet, a full rejuvenative program and fasting should help you rid your body of all the nasty poisons you've been ingesting and give you a new lease on life.'

'How much actual fasting will there be?'

'Let's not worry about that right now,' he suggested. 'We'll design the program around you, to suit your needs as we go along. Now because I'm a medical doctor first and foremost, you have nothing to worry about here at Elysian. You're in very safe hands.'

After the examination I was shown to my room, which was a little bungalow set apart from the rest of the building. It overlooked a somewhat unkempt swimming pool. Plant detritus floated on the surface and I could see sticks and all sorts of other rubbish on the bottom. My room was tidy, though, if a bit spare. Dr Goldman left me to settle in and unpack. I hadn't brought much – a few changes of clothes, my toiletry bag and some books. If you're one of those people who think they can make psychological assessments of others by what reading matter they find on bedside tables, it will, no doubt, fascinate you to know that I had with me: *The Catcher in The Rye* by J D Salinger, *Lost Horizon* by James Hilton, *Man's Search for Meaning* by Victor Frankl and a volume of Somerset Maugham's short stories. Make of that what you will.

As I was settling in the resident nurse came to see me. She was wearing a sort of nurse's outfit so she was either a nurse or a stripper. She took out a thermometer and a clipboard. Yep, definitely a nurse. Too bad . . .

'Why do I need my temperature taken now?' I asked.

'Oh, we like to monitor everyone as they go along. Fasting can be a taxing business, particularly when you've been living on artificial food and stimulants your whole life – the poisons that people slowly kill themselves with. Like cigarettes and tea and coffee.'

'You have tea and coffee here, don't you?' I asked.

'Of course not,' she said. 'And you know what? You won't even miss them.'

My heart sank. This was like telling a junkie he won't miss his smack. The nurse, who had introduced herself as Annie, left me with a 10-page questionnaire to fill in about everything from my bowel habits to what I dreamt at night. They were nothing if not thorough but some of the questions went beyond the bounds of privacy. For example, did they really have to know how many times a week I ejaculated and whether I had unsavoury, intrusive sexual fantasies? I wondered whether some weird cult really did run the place – were they trying to get inside my head so they could practise mind control?

After settling into my room I decided to have a look around before dinner. I wandered up the sloping lawn to the main building, which was kind of like a dormitory. Walking down the hallway, I could see people lying on beds, reading – it reminded me of some movie I'd seen set in a prison, actually – while a few others were gathered in a small lounge room watching the TV. This, I thought, looked promising. The person attached to the skeletal, bearded face I had seen at the window looked up, smiled and raised his arm to say hello.

'Welcome,' he said a bit feebly. 'I'm John.'

'Phil . . . hi.'

The others murmured greetings and I sat down. On the screen was footage of people in bathing suits throwing around a beach ball, all smiling. At first I thought that I'd stumbled into a porn session and that the frolicking on-screen was the preamble to some sort of orgy. But soon the folks featured all sat down at a long dinner table and started tucking into plate-loads of fresh fruit and veg, laughing and chatting as they did so.

'What is this?' I asked.

'Shhhh,' one girl said. 'This is an introduction to natural hygiene.'

'Natural hygiene?'

'Aren't you a hygienist? Isn't that why you're here?'

'I'm here to get healthy and detox but I don't know anything about natural hygiene. What is it?'

John reached over and handed me a small booklet, an introduction to natural hygiene, which sounded like something you might attend to in the loo. From a quick flick through it I gleaned that this was an extreme vegan dietary movement, one which looked like it had the potential to take all the joy out of life. Its central thesis is that humans should eat only raw foods, like fruit and veges and nuts and basically not much else. Comfort food was definitely out and tea and coffee were like arsenic, apparently.

'This sounds a bit extreme,' I said as the TV screen showed a close-up of someone chomping on a lettuce leaf with an orgasmic look on their face.

'Was it extreme in the Garden of Eden?' said John.

'Is it extreme for the mountain gorillas to eat the food God provides?' asked the girl. If these were jokes I didn't know the punchlines. My cousin Peter was right. The place was run by a cult made up of humourless, radical vegans. I was a bit thrown.

'Guys, I'd love to stay and chat but I think I better go before someone in this video starts having sex with that banana. I'll see you all at dinner.'

As I left the room I heard someone say, 'Dinner? Ha!', but I wasn't quite sure what that meant. I found out later that there was no communal dining, and when my meal arrived I could understand why because, basically, there was no bloody meal.

'Tell me this is not my dinner,' I said to Mrs Goldman, who had presented me with a glass of fruit juice.

'This is your sustenance. We have juice for a day or two and then we start the fast properly.'

'You mean the fast doesn't include juice?' I asked, crestfallen.

'Oh no,' she said. 'To purge your system of the filth you've been ingesting requires complete abstinence from everything but water.'

'Oh, good, I get water,' I said sarcastically. She left me to my juice and I sipped at it slowly, trying to make it last. It was thin juice, without any pulp, so I couldn't even chew it a bit on the way down. Sitting there, with the light fading and my tummy rumbling, something became very clear: I may have made a big mistake. I'd imagined that this was a place where healthy food would be laid on with a trowel except for a few days of juice fasting. I thought there'd be spas and massage and that sort of thing, but there didn't seem to be any evidence of that sort of activity at all. For the privilege of not eating I had paid $1500, which seemed a bit steep considering the fact that it was now obvious that that covered the room only. But maybe this is what I needed . . . I lay back on the bed and picked up *Lost Horizon* for some escapism.

Next morning my juice was served at 8 a.m. I was well and truly awake by then because I'd had a splitting headache since about 5 a.m. – the result, I guessed, of already going without my caffeine and tannin fixes for a whole evening. As I sat on the edge of the bed sipping the insipid libation, I watched a few of the other inmates perambulating slowly around the lawn. None of them looked too healthy actually, which was a bit of a worry since this was a health farm – sorry, 'sanitarium', as they insisted on calling it. After my juice, which I downed in about two seconds flat, I went out and sat on the lawn for a while, sunning myself. It was only day one but already time was starting to drag. I kept telling myself that this would be good for me and that I'd feel like a million dollars at the end of it all. No pain, no gain.

'Hang in there,' said John, the gaunt one, who wandered past and seemed to be reading my thoughts. 'Every day in every way you're getting better and better and better.'

Had he read that on a desk calendar or what?

'Sure,' I said. 'Feeling a bit peckish, though.'

'Oh, don't worry,' he said. 'It takes a while to correct and re-educate the body and the palate. But once you leave here you won't be able to eat what you ate before. You'll crave only raw, natural food . . . the way nature intended it.'

I went back to my room because in my increasingly famished state I was feeling more antisocial than usual. The hungrier I got, the grumpier I got, and I was not in a good mood when Dr Goldman did his rounds.

'How are you feeling?' he asked, peering into my eyes with a small but powerful torch.

'Well, I could eat the crotch out of a low-flying duck right now, but apart from that I'm fine,' I said.

'Yes, well, it gets worse before it gets better,' he offered. 'It's all part of the process.'

Easy for him to say. He had enough lard on him to last through an Antarctic winter, whereas I am naturally slim – there wasn't an ounce of excess fat on me. So what would happen to me if I went without food for too long, I wondered? I hadn't expected this extreme treatment at all. I thought I'd be eating wholemeal cookies and veggie pies, playing table tennis and walking in the woods. But this obviously wasn't that sort of health farm.

Later that day I attended the TV room and joined the others watching another crushingly boring video about dietary extremism. This time the subject matter was food combining for better digestion – riveting stuff. The food was squirrel tucker and the folks eating it all looked trim, tanned and completely insane, smiling madly over a few bean sprouts and chomping raw cashews as if they were tabs of acid. I went back to my room afterwards and felt very, very alone.

'Cheer up,' said nurse Annie when she brought me my evening fruit juice.

'I'd cheer up if you were serving a slice of pie with that,' I said. She laughed, at least, and left me lying on the bed, staring at the ceiling, thinking about food the way a sex addict might think about sex.

Over the next few days that's almost all I thought about. Food, not sex. Even the fact that I had a nurse coming to my room regularly had no impact, as prurient thought was out of the question. By the fourth day I was on water only.

'Are you sure this is safe?' I asked Dr Goldman.

'Fasting is safe and very beneficial,' he answered with certainty. I could smell food on the bugger's breath.

'How long will I be fasting for?'

'Oh, we'll wait and see,' he said. I rang my mother later that day, as I had promised to keep her informed of my progress. Knowing what a worrier she is, I played down the severity of the situation, said I felt fine and that I was sure it was doing me a power of good. But after that I phoned my Greek workmate, Cratis Hippocrates, at *The Gold Coast Bulletin*. He sounded worried when I told him what was going on.

'What you need is a good souvlaki,' he said.

'Souvlaki is in very short supply around here, mate,' I said. 'In fact these buggers don't believe in meat. They're all vegetarians.'

'Yeah, well, meat is a vegetable to us Greeks,' he said. 'Hey listen, are you gonna be okay down there? Maybe you should chuck it in and come home. You don't sound so hot. You want us to come down there and break you out?'

I said I'd give it a few more days and see how I felt, but I already knew how I felt: terrible. I was starting to hallucinate about food now and was getting weaker by the hour. I had to stop reading my Victor Frankl because I was starting to believe I knew how he felt in the concentration camp. And I understood why everyone else in the joint looked so shithouse. They were starving to death! But I needed sustenance, and the next day, weak as I was, I asked Mrs Goldman – who was starting to look and sound like an evil henchwoman from a James Bond movie – if I could go for a walk outside the grounds. She reluctantly agreed. I had in my mind's eye a recollection of that little shop not far up the road. I figured I could get there and back in under an hour and eat whatever stash of food I bought on the return lap. I was desperate.

I struggled along the largely deserted road, chafed by a chilly breeze, made it to the shop and bought myself two

Mars bars and a packet of Twisties. I didn't want to overdo it; I just wanted to get my blood sugar registering again. I shuffled back down the road to the sanitarium, munching as I went, and back in my room I cleaned my teeth thoroughly so that no-one would smell the chocolate on my breath. Instead of easing my hunger, though, all my indiscretion had given me was a sugar high, which made me even more ravenous. The next day I was so hungry I was virtually delirious. I wasn't quite as hungry as those Uruguayan rugby players who'd tucked into their buddies after that plane crash in the Andes, but I was close.

Meanwhile, I was starting to seriously suggest to the doctor, his wife, the nurse and anyone else who would listen that it was high time I ate something. I was getting weaker by the day and couldn't even muster the effort to shave in the morning, so I was now sporting a scrappy beard. The upside of that was that I thought I looked kind of like D H Lawrence, but then I remembered that the photograph of the famous author I based that on was taken not long before he died of consumption. The lack of nutrition was making me a wee bit more delusional than usual. But I was still rational enough to go to Dr Goldman and demand relief.

'Oh, but you are doing so well,' he said.

'Look, I'm sorry, but I've had enough,' I said. 'I need food and I need it now.'

He shrugged and said: 'If you insist. I'll get Mrs Goldman to prepare some vegetables.'

'Vegetables aren't going to cut it,' I said.

'But we have to re-introduce food slowly and carefully so your metabolism can adapt.' He didn't know about the Mars bars and the Twisties.

'Well, alright then,' I sulked. 'I guess that'll be okay. But could I have them cooked, if you don't mind?' I shuffled back to my room and was soon brought a dish of steamed potato and carrot. Luxury! I wolfed it down and spent the rest of the night dreaming about what I might eat next.

Next morning, after a piddling breakfast of fresh fruit – doled out very grudgingly, I might add – I went up to reception to discuss my meals for the day. I had a few more days of my stay to run and wanted to get my strength back. The Goldmans seemed to be preparing to go out.

'Talk to Annie, Mr Brown,' Mrs Goldman said, mildly annoyed. 'Unfortunately, we're going to be out most of the day in Sydney.'

That statement spurred me into a daring gambit. 'Well, would you mind if I went along for the ride?' I asked, but it was more of a demand really.

'But you haven't finished your program,' she said.

'Believe me, Mrs Goldman, I have finished my program. I won't be a bother. Where are you heading?'

'To Avalon to see some clients,' said Dr Goldman, who had come back inside after bringing the car around to the front of the building. It was a rather spiffy Jaguar. There's obviously money in starving people.

'Perfect,' I said. 'I'm heading for my aunt and uncle's place in Wahroonga, so you could drop me somewhere nearby. I'll just ring them first and tell them I will be a couple of days early.' I could have rung my cousin Peter to come and get me but he would have taken a while to get out here and I wanted an immediate escape. So, after ringing my Aunty Meg, who sounded worried — she had obviously been talking to Mum — I grabbed my bag and virtually forced my way into the back seat of the Goldmans' Jag. They seemed unnerved, but with liberation in sight I wasn't concerned about them any more.

It wasn't the most comfortable atmosphere on the drive into Sydney — in fact you could have cut the air with a knife for most of the way, but I didn't give a shit. I felt like a hostage who had taken charge of his captors. Natural hygiene — what a load of crap! Give me unnatural hygiene any day, I thought. Anyway, I'm sure the Goldmans ate what they wanted, unless their obesity was genetic, which I doubted.

Eventually we reached the leafy suburbs of the North Shore and I told them I'd get out near a train station. Aunty Meg and Uncle Maurice were expecting me at their home — I told them I'd catch a cab. I virtually threw myself out of the Goldmans' car and watched the Jag speed off.

'Bastards!'

I was pretty angry, but a few moments later my anger turned to joy at what I saw in front of me. There, just across the road, was a sign that seemed as attractive as an oasis mirage to a disoriented Bedouin. It declared, simply, 'Cakes'. I was immediately overwhelmed by an appetite more akin to lust than hunger. I rushed across the road, dodging traffic, and burst into the shop. The smell was heavenly and I put down my bag and surveyed the wonders before me . . . apple slices, neenish tarts, vanilla slices, lamingtons and cream buns that smelt as fresh as the ones I used to get in Grade One. I started ordering with élan, and didn't finish until I had filled three brown paper bags with goodies.

'Off to morning tea?' asked the lady behind the counter, a large woman in one of those foofy uniforms people in cake shops seem to wear.

'Um . . . yes,' I lied. 'Just having a few friends over.' I paid for the cakes and piled into a cab at the rank nearby.

'Gees, that lot smells good,' said the driver.

'Just drive,' I said.

'Well, it'll help if I know where I'm driving to,' he said.

'Chauvel Close, Wahroonga,' I said, spitting bits of coconut onto the dash.

'Hungry, mate?' the driver said as I scoffed another lamington and then pulled out a nice, moist piece of apple slice.

'Look, cabbie, between here and Chauvel Close I intend to eat all three of these bags of cakes, so excuse me if I don't feel too chatty while I'm at it.'

He looked at me sideways. 'Fair enough,' he said.

By the time we got there I'd finished the cakes. My aunt looked horrified when she saw me and took instant remedial action – that is, she put the kettle on.

'Your mother is very worried about you,' she said. 'You've lost a lot of weight. Would you like something to eat?'

'Oh yeah,' I said. I spent the next half-hour devouring

Saos, Scotch Finger biscuits and two peanut butter sandwiches, all washed down with copious cuppas. My tannin reserves were starting to top up again, thank God, but my blood sugar still had a way to go. After a little while all that food on an empty stomach gave me a stomach ache, and I retired to the spare room to lie down. I stayed that way, holding my belly and groaning, for the next few hours. I'm sure my aunt and uncle were sitting in the lounge room, doing their crosswords, shaking their heads. I repeated this cycle for days but never seemed to be able to eat enough. When I finally got back home to the Gold Coast after a long and gruelling bus trip, my mother was equally worried because I still looked wasted. She threatened to report the Elysian Sanitarium for criminal abuse of her eldest son.

The really galling part was when I caught up with Mark, the friend who had recommended the place. I told him we'd do a debriefing over a cheap Mexican meal, and when we sat down he looked vaguely guilty.

'Well, it's not your fault,' I said. 'It was that dickhead who recommended it to you that you should blame.'

'Yes, but I feel terrible,' he said. 'Because he told me about two health farms, one which he recommended and the other which he tried and checked out of on his third day.'

'And?'

'Well, I got them mixed up,' he said.

'You are kidding me?' I said. 'You mean I went to the wrong one? You've got to be bloody joking.'

'But you look well,' he said, grasping at straws.

'Yeah, right,' I said, turning to the waitress. 'Bring me another taco would you, luv,' I barked. 'No, wait . . . better make that a double.'

Group Grope

He chewed the stem of his pipe and fixed me with a deep, meaningful look. 'So you're angry?'

'No, Lionel, I'm not angry,' I said.

'It's called denial.'

'Is it?'

'You're angry that I suggest you're angry?'

'Not really.'

'Well, I'm sensing anger.'

'Well, I probably will get angry, I suppose, if you keep talking about how angry I am. That will make you happy, will it?'

'Ah,' he said sucking at the unlit pipe. 'And is this a new anger or an old anger?'

As a therapy, Transaction Analysis seemed self-fulfilling because by the time I finished a session with Lionel I'd be so pissed off that I'd have to book in for another session to deal with the anger. Pretty good business development technique, if you ask me.

Group Grope

I'd been going to Lionel for a few weeks. He was the latest dalliance in my quest for wellbeing at a time in my life when I was, well, *still* searching for answers – always a danger, because you'll come across people who think they have them. Terri, an acquaintance I had met at yoga, suggested that the answer to my unease was psychotherapy and that I consult Lionel.

I hadn't been very successful at yoga. For a start, the classes were held in a room just above the main street in Southport – I found the traffic noise disconcerting, and couldn't concentrate. Also, I wasn't supple enough to do half the positions, and spent most of my lessons grunting and groaning as I attempted to extend bits that didn't want to be extended.

'You're so into your own head,' said Terri after one class. 'You need to reprogram your brain, do something to quieten down all that mental and emotional chatter.'

'Really,' I said. 'So do you have some Valium on you?'

'You don't need Valium. You should just go and see this guy I've been to, Lionel. He's brilliant – very intuitive, very grounded.'

I don't think I've ever really worked out what 'grounded' means.

Lionel's therapy technique, as I soon found out, seemed to include a mish-mash of psychobabble but its foundation was Transactional Analysis, which was in vogue at the time, in the self-indulgent 1980s. 'TA', as those in the know called it, had been promulgated by Eric Berne, the author of *Games People Play* and *What Do You Say After You Say Hello?*

Thomas Harris was another TA guru and the author of *I'm OK – You're OK*. I had skimmed the latter in the reading frenzy that I was going through at that time. I was reading anything and everything to do with health, wellbeing and spirituality, and was becoming increasingly confused in the process. TA was all about reconciling and 'stroking' the various components of the psyche, which sounded pretty simple compared to some of the other claptrap I'd come across. The fact that we're all okay seemed an attractive proposition as long as you didn't think about it too much. Ponder it for too long and you might find yourself asking – was Pol Pot okay? Or Ted Bundy?

Though Lionel could be frustrating at times, he was a very convincing guy, a bit of a Svengali really. He made you think you were discovering amazingly revelatory things about yourself in his sessions – things that would free you up spiritually, emotionally and even financially. Looking back, a lot of the New Age stuff in the 1980s seemed to have monetary success as its goal ...

Lionel insisted on carrying out his sessions sitting in beanbags, which was a bit weird. It's hard to concentrate when a mountain of beans is constantly shifting under your bum but he insisted that beanbags were great levellers. Assuming he was as uncomfortable as I was, perhaps he was right.

One of the things I noticed about him was that whenever I went to see him, there were attractive young women coming out of a session or waiting to go in after me. Maybe analysing hornbags was his speciality? Once, when I arrived early for an appointment, a girl in a matching cheesecloth skirt and blouse rushed out past me while I was in the waiting room. She had come out of Lionel's room and seemed to be doing up her blouse, which made me raise an eyebrow at the time. But I thought, 'Nah.'

Anyway, after a couple of months the novelty of this head-shrinking well and truly wore off, and I announced to Lionel that I was going to give up therapy because I couldn't afford it (it was $50 a session, which was a lot of money back then, to me at least). This was partly true, though the main reason was that I felt I was just going round in ever-decreasing circles. I was gullible but not that gullible.

'So you're cured, are you?' Lionel said sarcastically when I told him.

'I don't know about cured.'

'Neither do I,' he said and stared at me for a few seconds. 'If we're going to wind up our sessions I want you to do two things for me.'

'Such as?' I asked suspiciously.

'I want you to read this book and come to a group therapy session this weekend.' He passed me *If You Meet the Buddha On the Road, Kill Him!* by Sheldon Kopp, a book about the pilgrimage of psychotherapy that was popular at that time.

'Poor old Buddha, what the hell did he do to deserve this?' I said. 'I really don't know about this group thing. I'm just not into groups.'

'Well, just come for the Saturday session and see what you think. It's on me.' A freebie is always good, even if it is only for group therapy. And there was always the chance that I might get a date out of it if nothing else.

That Saturday I turned up for the all-day seminar called *Getting to Know Your Adult-Parent-Child*. TA broke everyone down into these ego states and contended that the dynamic between them was what motivated the way we behave. That didn't sound too unreasonable. There were about 20 people in Lionel's office, which he had expanded by opening up a concertina partition. We all sat on beanbags and cushions. The group was predominantly female — there were only four blokes, counting me.

The morning session was spent with everyone spilling their guts at the behest of Lionel, who reckoned he was trying to 'break down the barriers' and get everyone loosened up a bit. He'd write stuff up on huge sheets of butcher's paper that he had on a stand out front. There was a lot of scribbling about how we were feeling, what we were feeling, who we were feeling it about.

'I want to ask you how you are feeling and what you want to say to the group, Tom,' Lionel asked one of the other guys, who was sitting there stony-faced. 'Tom?'

'I'm feeling like a real dickhead,' said Tom.

'And what do you want to say to the group?'

'I want to say "fuck you".'

Not nice. But Lionel seemed pleased with that.

'What about you, Vivien?'

'I'm feeling vulnerable,' she said. 'Very vulnerable but I also feel like I want to reach out to someone, to reach out and really connect with someone.'

I felt the urge to huddle in the far corner of the room.

'That's beautiful,' said Lionel. 'That's really beautiful, and sometime today we hope we can create a safe space where you can do that.'

Where's a bucket when you need one?

Encouraged by this twaddle, other people began spewing up their innermost thoughts. They were doing it to a bunch of strangers with alarming ease. This thing was turning positively Californian.

My outpouring was very brief and very restrained. I think I said something like: 'I'm only here because Lionel wouldn't let me drop therapy without coming here for the day.'

'Phil has some issues that he isn't dealing with, but that's okay too,' said Lionel coolly, but I could see he was steamed up. 'As the day progresses he might discover what some of them are.' I looked at my watch and groaned.

Brad, one of the other blokes there, was less reticent. He was there with his girlfriend and neither of them looked liked they'd had a bath for quite a while. They were up for the weekend from Mullumbimby and they had clung to each other like limpets since we first sat down. Brad was quite verbal when it came to expressing his inner child, you might say, and this inner child just wouldn't shut up.

After one of Brad's lengthy verbal ejaculations, Lionel – nodding in a sagely fashion and sucking on his unlit pipe – said: 'Well, that's beautiful, Brad. Now how to deal with that in your relationship? How do you think Cindy can comfort you?'

Cindy piped up then. 'I like to help Brad feed his inner child by holding him in my arms like a baby with my breast in his mouth,' she said. 'Sometimes he'll do that for ages, just lying there, suckling.'

I didn't know where to look. Part of me wanted to shout out, 'Way to go, Brad!', while another part of me squirmed with embarrassment. I mean, did we really need to know that? Everyone else nodded and smiled like subjects under hypnosis. I looked up at the wall clock then and saw that it was nearly noon. I started praying for the session to end before someone started talking about pleasuring themselves.

We broke for lunch, which was put out on a couple of small tables at the back of the room. There were alfalfa sprout sandwiches, some sort of fried vegetable dumplings, a few carrot sticks and other vegetarian treats — hardly the sort of thing to sustain a grown man through an afternoon session with Lionel and his merry band. I chewed on one of the sprout sangers — it tasted like chaff. I washed it down with a cup of peppermint tea, which was all that was on offer besides water.

'I'd give my left nut for a short black,' I joked, but that didn't seem to go down so well.

'So what do you do?' one girl asked. I didn't know what to say at first because I was taken aback by a sour odour that seemed to arrive with her. Body odour, that is. I've never understood what hippies have against bathing. And would it kill them to use some roll-on deodorant?

'I'm a journalist,' I said.

She sort of turned her nose up, which was a bit rich since I was the one who should have been doing that.

'Oh,' she said. 'That must be weird.'

'I don't know about weird,' I said. 'But it sure beats working for a living. What about you?'

'I just live,' she said. 'That's it. I just live, you know what I mean?'

'Living's good,' I said. 'Living is very acceptable. It's better than the alternative.'

Bloody nutter, I thought, what about getting a job? Heck, all of a sudden I was channelling my old man. I hadn't been looking forward to the afternoon session but when Lionel came back into the room, reeking of Amphora – proof that he did actually sometimes light that pipe of his – I was pleased. I wasn't sure how much more chit-chat I could manage with these flakes.

As we sat down again, rustling in our beanbags, listing this way and that, I had the urge to flee almost immediately – but Lionel had already begun talking, and to do a runner now would draw the sort of attention I definitely didn't want. And if I'd thought the morning session was emotionally confronting, well the afternoon's session left it for dead. I mean, personally I'm in favour of people hanging on to their deep dark secrets and sexual fantasies. They're not really secrets or fantasies any more when they're in the public domain. I favour an uptight, restrained society. Victorian England has always seemed a good model to me, but these people had swallowed the whole Californian ideal of unburdening oneself endlessly in the search for enlightenment.

Some of the girls were being especially candid. A lass called

Toni, one of the few who didn't look 'alternative' – she wore square clothes and thickish glasses – completely shocked me with a fantasy about making love with a gorilla. I couldn't believe my ears, and wanted to shout: 'Please, make her stop!' This was a bit much even for Lionel, who moved her fantasy along pretty quickly for fear it would turn nastier than it already was.

Everyone else seemed normal compared to that. Sally, another of the hippie chicks there, revealed that she was having sexual thoughts about several blokes in the room. I guess I must have had tickets on myself back then because I looked out the window terrified that she might mean me. She wasn't exactly the most attractive person, and her arms were hairier than your average Greek male's.

Lionel, though he looked serious and solemn, really seemed to enjoy most of these revelations, and encouraged the speakers to go further each time. He even hugged people occasionally – though not the blokes, I noticed, and I can't blame him for being prejudiced because some of these fruitcakes were pretty foxy fruitcakes. I became increasingly uncomfortable, though, as the afternoon wore on, and couldn't quite work out where this was all leading. The structured TA therapy which he'd shown us by way of a diagram he'd scribbled at the beginning of the day seemed to have been abandoned for a sort of freewheeling encounter session. I started seeing flashbacks from the movie *Woodstock*.

What had started out as a fairly innocuous experience now seemed almost sinister. Lionel was starting to look more and more like Charles Manson to me and these chicks could have been the Family. Helter Skelter is upon us again, I thought. This is the sort of stuff that runs through your mind during severe caffeine withdrawal.

When the session finally came to an end, with much hugging and some tears, I was fazed out completely. When I realised Lionel was done, I was more enthusiastic than I had been all day. A wave of immense relief washed over me. One of the girls – Julie, I think her name was – who was wearing a prayer shirt with nothing under it, came up and asked me what I thought of the whole thing.

'Well, to tell you the truth, it was all a bit daunting for me,' I said. 'Way too touchy-feely.'

'Far out,' she said and then tried to hug me. I sidestepped her and decided to high-tail it out of there before the call for the group hug went up.

I ran into Terri in Southport the following week.

'You must come over to a party I'm having this weekend,' she said. 'There'll be some really interesting people there.'

'I hate interesting people,' I said. 'I met enough interesting people last weekend at Lionel's seminar. Never again.'

'Oh, I forgot you were seeing Lionel,' she said. 'He is so stuck in a rut with all that TA stuff.'

'But you're the one who suggested I go and see him.'

'Yes, yes, I remember, but I don't buy that TA stuff any more,' she said.

'But it was only a couple of months ago.'

'A lot can happen in a couple of months if you follow the *I Ching*. Anyway, Lionel is only in it for the sex.'

'The what?'

'Well, he has sex with all his patients,' she said. 'Didn't you know that?'

'He never had sex with me,' I said. I may have been joking but I was surprised. Make that shocked!

'With all his women patients, obviously, is what I mean,' she said. 'He's a shocker. Tried to jump my bones once while I was sitting in one of those damn beanbags. Terrible things . . . you can't get up out of them fast enough. Ugh. No thank you.'

'You're saying he has sex with women . . . in his rooms?'

'Absolutely,' she said.

'Bastard,' I said.

'Exactly.'

'Lucky bastard, I mean.'

She punched me, hard.

What a Bummer

I was cruising along the Gold Coast Highway looking for a parking spot when I found one out front of the Oriental Bath House. I wondered if anybody ever actually went there for a bath? If someone I knew had been driving past Mermaid Beach at that time, on that day, they might have made a very wrong assumption about my destination. I slammed the car door, looked around somewhat furtively and then walked a hundred metres south. The bath house was situated in a snazzy new building but I was heading for a dowdy little block of shops next door – a remnant of the 1950s from the look of it, when Mermaid Beach was just one of a string of relatively sleepy seaside villages. The front shop of this down-at-heel complex was a little organic food store selling the sort of stuff that only budgies should eat along with various other alternative products. The smell of incense leaked through the open door and hung in the air.

'We're behind the organic produce store,' I'd been told

by the receptionist. 'Just walk down the lane beside it for 50 feet or so and you'll come to a door on your left.'

The lane was a bit scuzzy, which was somewhat off-putting. It hadn't been hosed or swept in a while but I was definitely on the right track because on a glass door there was a sign:

'Colonic Irrigation Clinic – Please Enter'.

Now you could interpret that in a couple of ways, I thought as I pushed open the door and went into a small, freezing waiting room. It was so cold in there that condensation had formed on the windows due to the heat and humidity outside. It was like being in one of those Bangkok tailor shops where you go just to get out of the muggy atmosphere rather than to have a suit made – although once you're in one, you're trapped, and will soon be measured to within an inch of your life.

Of course this wasn't Bangkok, it was definitely no tailor shop and I was already starting to feel like I didn't really want to be here. I had been talked into this therapeutic escapade over dinner one night at Tamari Bistro in Surfers Paradise. Colonic irrigation is not the sort of thing you really want to be talking about over dinner but my friend Ari's very persistent wife, Elaine – an aficionado of New Age health treatments – wouldn't let the subject drop.

'You really shouldn't eat red meat,' she said as I tucked into my veal parmigiana.

'Veal isn't red meat, is it?' I said. 'It's more sort of deep pink.'

'Any meat will clog you up,' she said. 'What, you want bowel cancer, do you?'

'I don't think anybody wants bowel cancer,' I said. 'But a bit of red meat now and then can't hurt. Besides, Ari is eating it too.' She looked at her husband as he cut his veal with the precision of a surgeon.

'He's a lost cause,' she said, shaking her head. 'Anyway, if you do eat red meat regularly, you should also have regular colonic irrigation.' Ari flinched at the mention.

'Oh, no no no,' I said. 'No way. I let nature take its course when it comes to my innards.'

'But you're eating red meat and that's not natural, that's not letting nature take its course,' Elaine insisted. 'Nature's course is eating fruit and vegetables and nuts and herbs . . . the things that God meant us to eat.'

'If God didn't intend us to eat meat, then why did He create butchers?' I reasoned. She scowled. 'I have a high colonic once a month,' she declared in an overloud voice. Several diners looked over, and Ari and I hunched over our plates.

'What about you, Ari? Have you tried colonic irrigation?' I asked.

He nodded sheepishly. 'She makes me go.'

'It gets rid of all the toxins,' Elaine persisted. 'The amount of coffee you guys drink and the crap you eat, you should be going for one every damn day.' Now that *did* sound extreme.

'There'd be nothing left of us if we did,' I laughed and forked down another piece of immature cow. Actually I didn't really know much about colonic irrigation, although the principle sounded pretty self-evident. And in the Eighties everybody on the Gold Coast seemed to be doing it... along with sensory deprivation float-tanks and Reiki and a host of other wacky therapies. When all this is happening around you, after a while you start to weaken and think there might be something in it.

I'd been feeling a little off-colour lately, too, and had tried various naturopathic cures for my self-diagnosed neurasthenia. I tried to pep myself up by drinking about 10 flat whites a day at Tamari Bistro, where I spent half my time. I was working as a freelance journalist and the café was my 'field office'. Ari and Elaine were regulars there too, which is how we got friendly. She was forgoing the coffee nowadays for herbal tea and kept nagging me about doing the same but herbal tea has always made me gag. Chamomile... yuk! But she wouldn't let up about this colonic irrigation business.

'What, have you got shares in the joint?' I asked her one day after another ear-bashing on the subject.

'No, but I wish I did because it's going to be big business in the future,' she said. 'Look, here's a card for Gunther's clinic. Just go along and try it once. You'll feel so much better.'

'Better than what?' I asked and she narrowed her eyes.

'Do yourself a favour for a change,' she said.

Though the actual physical concept was pretty repugnant to me, I must admit the idea of detoxification seemed vaguely attractive. I mean, if you could get all the crap out of your body – literally – in just one go, that would be a hell of a lot easier than all these detox diets. They take weeks, months. But this would be – *whooshka!* – so quick and easy . . . wouldn't it? Eventually I caved in and made an appointment to see Gunther. I never really got too experimental with drugs when I was young, apart from the spliffs and bongs that went with being a surfie and were compulsory in student share-housing. But I did have something of a penchant for experimenting with treatments I thought might make me feel better. That quest had already taken me down some weird paths, on which I'd met some odd people, but by now weird paths and odd people were starting to seem normal to me. If I kept going the way I was going, eventually I would get around to trying them all.

So I sat in Gunther's chilly, miniscule waiting room, waiting. No-one was about so I rang the small bell on the counter and a bespectacled, bearded face peered from between black curtains drawn across a narrow doorway. Was this the ghost of John Lennon?

'I'm sorry, my receptionist iss not here juss now, I be wiss you in a moment,' he said in a German accent. 'Make yourself comfortable.'

Comfortable? Yeah right. Comfortable was the one thing I did not feel, and I shifted in my seat nervously as I flicked through a *National Geographic*. I had settled into reading an article about orang-utans – who reminded me of a couple of the editors I'd worked for – when the curtains opened again and a very large, sweaty man was ushered out from behind them. He got caught in them momentarily and fought to get free, and then, embarrassed, rushed past me like a hippo on the trot.

'Goodbye, see you nexx month,' Gunther said as the door swung shut. Then he looked at me with a scary sort of smile. My first thought was to flee because I was having one of those moments you have in some reeking public toilet when you're busting to go but the cubicles are full. Then some unkempt, oversized individual emerges from one cubicle, still hitching up his daks, and you have to make a crucial decision: do I really want to go where that man has gone before? Do I really want to sit on the same seat, breathe the same air? How badly do I really want to go? And in this instance I asked myself — would I be serviced today with the same equipment that has just serviced the fat guy? Would apparatus that has just touched his now touch mine? The thought was too heinous to even consider.

'I'm Gunther,' the practitioner then said, breaking my dour reverie, formalising the meeting and offering me his hand — a wet hand. He had presumably just washed them after his last client. Couldn't he have dried them, too? Would that have been too much to ask? I mean, what if the germs were still on them, swimming in the viscous surface of the hand, post-wash? Had he even used antiseptic soap?

'You look tense,' Gunther said. 'Juss relax and I vill be wiss you in a few moments.'

I took my hand back and looked at it. It's moments like these when you know you should always carry moist towelettes everywhere you go — and I mean everywhere. I wiped the hand on the back of my trousers and made a mental note not to put it anywhere near my face until I had got home and rinsed it in some industrial-strength Dettol.

A few minutes later Gunther's head appeared through the curtains again.

'Come ziss way, please, Phil,' he said. I felt like I was going behind the curtains into one of those adult bookshops. Not that I had ever been into one. But there was nothing saucy behind the curtains here – just a treatment room and a none too inspiring one at that. It was a small space – way too cramped for my liking. My claustrophobia immediately kicked in. I've always had a fear of enclosed spaces, which is probably why I'm scared of flying and why those float-tanks have never really appealed to me. I also find it difficult to watch movies about submarines, and once had a panic attack while watching *Das Boot*. To be fair, there were windows but they were heavily curtained, presumably so nobody would perve through them at Gunther's clients; though I can't imagine anyone getting their jollies from watching a colonic irrigation in progress. But then again, there are some sick puppies out there.

'So, you are familiar with ze therapy?' Gunther asked.

'Sort of,' I said. 'I mean, I get the general idea.'

'Yes, well, ze colon picks up a lot of poison and noxious debris because of ze vay ve are eating nowadays, and since ve get our nutrients from food ve also get our toxins from it too.'

I nodded.

'Und zo much of vot ve ingest now has not got nutritional value at all. Tea, coffee, junk food. Ziss all leads to autointoxication und an accumulation of harmful material in ze colon.'

I nodded again.

'Ackchewally, colon irrigation or colonic hydrotherapy goes back to ancient Egypt, you know, but wasn't really revived in zer West until ze larse century. Now it is being recognised again, which is good, ja?'

I nodded a third time.

'Do you haff any questions about ze procedure?'

'Yes,' I said. 'How long will it take?'

'Don't be so vorried, it vill only take about 45 minutes. Have you been eating ze light diet for the past day or so ass ve suggest?'

'Oh yes,' I said. 'Minestrone, minestrone and more minestrone. And the odd Salada.'

'Zer gutt. Now, for your treatment you will lay down and ve vill introduce varm, purified water vich vill help to force out zer nasty material sroo ze evacuation tube. Please take your close off an put ziss robe on.' He handed me one of those back-to-front hospital gowns. I put it on the wrong way around, exposing my wedding tackle. Not a good look.

'No, it goes ze ozzer way around,' he said. I slipped my arms into the holes again and covered my front, leaving my bum exposed to the breeze from the air conditioner above. The robe seemed unnecessary, but maybe it made Gunther feel more like a medico.

'Now you juss get up on ze bench, breeze deeply und relax. Put your feet in here and lie back.'

I got up onto the bench and he guided my ankles into stirrups that looked like they were set up for some serious gynaecological event. He fiddled around with some equipment and I tried to relax, but became tenser second by second. What the hell was I doing in this demeaning position? I asked myself. I knew on one level that it was all supposed to be doing me a power of good, but on another level it was just plain humiliating. Degrading. And . . .

'What the hell!!!!'

'You muss relax,' he insisted as he inserted a hose down where the sun don't shine.

As the probe was secured, I gulped and looked at the ceiling, mortified. If this wasn't the most humiliating moment in my life, it was close.

'Oh, please relax,' he insisted again. 'You must not fight it.' Wasn't that what torturers said as they administered truth serum or attached electrodes to your whatsits?

I wanted to say: 'It's pretty hard to relax when you're being violated by a complete stranger,' but instead merely whimpered, 'Okay, I'll try. But I'm not very good with medical procedures. I'm a bit squeamish. I faint when I have a blood test.'

'You vill be fine,' he said. 'Juss lie back and let everything flow.'

Speaking of flowing, the water started up now and I was experiencing a ticklish feeling and suction, which was quite unnerving. I lay back and tried to think of England. I felt like I had been attached to some succubus that was draining the life force from me, an alien force that would turn me into a human husk within minutes – all for the sake of getting rid of a few toxins.

'How long did you say this would take?' I asked again in the humble tones the degraded uses to his degrader.

'Forty-five minutes, possibly an hour if zere iss a lot to clean out,' he said.

'Bugger me dead,' I said, without meaning to be Freudian.

'Vee haff to clean ze colon properly,' he said. 'Look, you can see ze toxins coming out already.'

But I could not look. I did not want to look. I did not want to watch this invasion of my bodily sanctuary. It was horrible! I felt like a moray eel had bitten me on the bum, held on and was now sucking the life out of me. Meanwhile the pump chugged away like the *African Queen* and I tried desperately to drift off, to distract myself. Because of the way I was lying, I tried to imagine I was an astronaut — and not one of the ones barbecued before take-off — fit and confident and heading for outer space with every expectation of a safe return. There I was, secure in my vast suit, my face hidden behind the bubble of my helmet. I could hear, from the depths of my imagination, David Bowie cranking up a bit of 'Space Oddity'. Major Tom felt pretty forlorn and abandoned, adrift in the cosmic void — and who could blame him? Imagine being up there for weeks, scared out of your wits, wondering whether you would ever return, defecating in your own clothing . . . no way!

Anyway, I was not in outer space, I was in a shabby little room in Mermaid Beach, next door to a brothel, having my bowel sucked dry by a guy who sounded like an extra on *Hogan's Heroes*. Mind you, he at least had the decency to vacate the room for a while during the procedure, leaving me to my own private ignominy. I lay there watching the ceiling and listening to the New Age soundtrack he'd put on. Oh no – whales again! The whale songs – or was it the sounds of them being harpooned? – were like Chinese water-torture drips.

I gazed around the room and focused on the fact that it was decidedly grubby. Now this is not the sort of place you want grubby. This is the sort of place that needs to be so clean you can eat off the toilet seat. This sort of place should have several air locks before entry and everyone should have been hosed down and be wearing germ-proof suits and gloves and shoe coverings and hermetically-sealed headgear. There should be no mould on the ceiling, no condensation on the windows, no musty smell, and the practitioner should not greet his patients with wet hands after playing with someone else's bum.

I felt the urge to get up but couldn't, being still hooked up to the evil apparatus. I caught a glimpse of the tubing and thought I saw part of my entrails being sucked out to be whisked away down some dirty drain. And that was when I snapped.

'Gunther!' I shouted. 'Gunther! Could you please come in here right now!'

'Vot is ze problem?' he asked sticking his head through the curtain the way Eric used to do on *The Morecambe and Wise Show*.

'I'm sorry,' I said. 'You'll have to unhook me. I can't do this.'

'You need to relax,' he said. 'Juss lie back and relax.'

'No, I'm sorry,' I said. 'I'm not doing that. You'll have to turn this infernal contraption off and unhook me immediately.'

'You are serious?' he asked. 'Zare is still 40 minutes of ze treatment left.' Was I sure I wanted to stop it? Did the prisoners in the dungeons at Gestapo headquarters mean it when they said they'd had enough interrogation? I meant what I said and insisted that he remove the hose from my behind so I could get the hell out of there and take what was left of my toxins with me.

He seemed rather annoyed by this treatment interruptus, but his feelings weren't high on my list of things to consider at that moment.

I got up, took off my back-to-front gown, dressed quickly and went back outside to the small counter where, guiltily, I insisted on paying the full price. He didn't argue about that.

'I'm sorry I haff to charge you for the whole session,' he said, though he obviously wasn't.

'That's okay,' I said. 'I don't mind.' I just wanted to be out of there. But though the treatment was over, I could still feel the effect – as if there was some phantom still sucking at me.

I got out of there and back on the street. As I was getting into my car, someone I knew drove past and tooted. I waved as I was getting in and suddenly thought: they think I've been to the brothel. I mean, I was parked right out front after all. But what the hell.

A week later, while slurping my third flat white and chomping on a pastry at Tamari, Elaine turned up. 'So how was your first colonic?' she asked.

I shook my head. 'Colonic irrigation is not for me,' I said.

'Oh, you big sissy,' she said. 'Colonic irrigation is for everyone. You must feel better after your treatment.'

'I didn't finish the treatment.'

'Oh, that's a shame,' she said. 'Well, you'll just have to go back and have another one.'

'No way,' I said. 'As far as I'm concerned, he can stick his colonic irrigation up his arse.'

Me of Little Faith

My friend Mary was always looking for the next big thing in gurus and off-beat treatments. She was constantly trying to get me involved in her latest fad as well, particularly since her husband wasn't the slightest bit interested. Whenever I turned up at their place she had a new thing going. I remember lobbing in one night to find that she had just discovered the mystical branch of Islam.

'I'm into Sufi,' she declared. I looked at her husband, Bob, a raging cynic, to gauge his reaction.

'I'm into goofy,' he said, deadpan. Mind you, the Sufism bug didn't last long with Mary, particularly because there really weren't any Sufi mystics around on the Gold Coast at that time, so it was hard for her to get any first-hand experience. By the time I visited again a few weeks later she had changed tack completely, and was into Filipino faith healing. She had somehow met this healer, Felipe Cruz, at a party and had claimed him as her new messiah.

'He is, of course, a fake,' Bob said.

'You wouldn't know,' Mary said. 'You're so closed to everything. You just smoke your weed and watch the world go by, don't you?'

'Oh, that reminds me,' said Bob, who put his guitar down and proceeded to roll himself a joint. Mary went over and closed the curtains.

'So what does this Felipe Cruz guy actually do?' I asked.

'He's a psychic surgeon,' she said. 'He removes diseased parts and cleanses the body ... so that it can heal. You should have seen all the stuff he dragged out of me. What a mess! It's all done without anaesthetic and his patients don't feel a thing. I've had a couple of treatments. It's really quite amazing.'

I looked at Bob, who had his own theory on this of course.

'What he actually — does,' Bob said, through half-held breath after inhaling some marijuana smoke, 'is rip people off. The stuff he supposedly removes from people is just chicken guts. It's so obvious: the whole thing is a total fraud.'

'Well, I felt a lot better after my treatment, so that proves something,' Mary said.

'It just proves there was nothing wrong with you in the first place,' said Bob. 'The only thing he removed from you was the money from your wallet.'

'I've seen these Filipino faith healers on TV,' I said. These healers, who practise what is known as psychic surgery, have been popular in the Philippines since the 1940s, and in the 1980s they went out into the world to spread their contentious practice. This method of healing people by apparently dragging diseased entrails from them through a sort of psychokinesis has been debunked as a hoax countless times, but that didn't seem to stop the proliferation of the faith healers. They were like modern shamen tapping into people's superstitious nature. They operated under the umbrella of Christianity but were really a part of more pagan traditions. There had been a recent exposé of them on one of the early evening current-affairs shows. People had been flocking to them from all over the world, many claiming miracle cures, which hadn't been proven or comprehensively debunked for that matter. I mean, how do you debunk faith? On TV they showed footage of one of these alleged charlatans dragging all sorts of bloody entrails from somebody and then declaring them cured. The patient looked very pleased.

'You should do a story on Felipe,' Mary said. 'He's really an amazing man.'

'What I find amazing,' said Bob, 'is that you've been sucked in by him.'

'Ye of little faith,' said Mary dismissively.

A couple of days later she phoned me to ask if I wanted to meet this Cruz guy for a free treatment, with a view to writing a story on him for one of the tacky magazines I contributed to at the time.

'I'm sure he can help you with your tummy troubles,' she insisted. 'It can't hurt, can it?'

'No, I guess not,' I agreed. My duodenal ulcer seemed to be making a comeback, which was causing me quite a bit of discomfort. I was living mostly on cracker biscuits and liquid antacid at this stage. My natural curiosity and my desperation made me agree to have a session.

'Can you come on Wednesday morning?'

I put it in my diary and turned up at the address she'd given me at the appointed time on the appointed day. It was a swanky address in a broad boulevard in one of those flash fake-canal estates that were then spreading insidiously into the landscape beyond Surfers Paradise. The front of the house was immaculate – not a blade of grass out of place and not a leaf in sight. There was some minimalist topiary and two shiny, black Mercedes-Benz in the wide driveway. I went to the front door, which was adorned with a crucifix just above a heavy brass knocker. A Filipino maid answered it and ushered me into a small room which might have been designed as a study but had now obviously been designated as the waiting room. It was full and that was surprising – only because everything had seemed so spare outside.

From the front the house seemed almost deserted, except for the cars in the driveway, but in here there was a madding crowd. Mary was supposed to be meeting me, but after quickly scanning the faces in the room I realised she wasn't there yet. The maid suggested I sit down. I wasn't too keen but I did as I was told and joined the throng. This was a depressing experience because everyone in there seemed to be maimed in some way. Being among sick people for any length of time is not good for a hypochondriac. I sat there and tried not to look at anyone. By the time the maid came back in I was thinking of doing a runner.

'Felipe will see you now,' she said. Some of the patients looked daggers at me then because it was pretty obvious that the healer was seeing me ahead of people who had already been waiting, I knew not how long. I guess that's one of the benefits of being a journalist – you can queue-jump at your local Filipino faith healer. I was led down a shag-carpeted hallway and into another small room to meet Felipe Cruz, who greeted me with an overly firm handshake. He had caught me unawares, though, by sticking his hand out before I was ready, and he was so quick off the mark that I only managed to get the tops of my fingers into his iron grip. So I couldn't return the firm greeting with the appropriate macho squeeze, which annoyed me. It's a guy thing.

'Welcome, welcome,' he said.

'Hello, nice to meet you,' I said, distracted from his visage momentarily by what sat above it – one of the thickest heads of hair I have ever seen, a virtual black helmet, a glistening mass held together by a substance that smelled suspiciously like Brylcreem. If you're old enough to remember the Brylcreem ads, you'll recall the catch-phrase, 'a little dab'll do ya', but this guy must have laid it on with a trowel. I hadn't seen Brylcreem on the shelves since I was a kid but maybe they still sold it in the Philippines. He looked like Elvis Presley.

Then I took in the room like a private detective trying to sum everything up in a few moments. There was the obligatory crucifix on the wall – Filipinos are, for the most part, devout Catholics – and a few pictures hanging nearby, one of Jesus with the sacred heart glowing in his chest, another of the Holy Mother, looking suitably radiant with a halo framing her head, and yet another of the Holy Family. Some of these psychic surgeons claim to be guided by saints and even by the Holy Spirit itself.

In the middle of the room was a massage table with a waterproof cover. Nearby stood a small table with a dish full of cotton wool swabs, a small stainless steel surgical tray and some sort of antiseptic – you could smell it in the room – in a small bottle. On the ground nearby was a bucket. All the mod cons of a medical field unit in the Crimea.

'Are you Catolik?' he asked.

'Yes,' I said.

'Do you beleef?'

'Well, kind of,' I said.

'We shall see,' he said. I had a sudden flashback to that running joke in Monty Python about the Spanish Inquisition. (You know the one: 'Nobody expects the Spanish Inquisition', they say, before apprehending their next victim.) Felipe sounded like some character ready to torture the truth out of me, the hapless heretic.

He asked what was wrong with me, and I told him I'd had some tummy troubles and was feeling generally run down. This wasn't very dramatic, and I felt like I really was there on false pretences – though I was keen to experience whatever it was that he did.

'Please take off you shirt and shoes and lie on dee table.'

I did as I was told, facing downwards with my head in

that little hole they have in massage tables that enables you to study the shag pile while you're being pummelled.

'No, please lie on you back,' he said, so I flipped over and stared at the ceiling.

'Will this hurt?' I asked.

'No, it only hurt me,' he said.

'Really? How come?'

'Only that it drain me, my energy . . . you see?'

'I think so.'

'Okay, you lie quiet now and we begin.'

He began prodding my abdomen with both hands. They were quite cold and gave me a start. Aren't you supposed to rub them to warm up before this sort of thing? He prodded, gently at first and then quite hard, so hard eventually that I started uttering little grunts each time he'd push into me. He stopped doing that for a moment, then walked around the table and started prodding again. This routine went on for a little while.

'Anything yet?' I asked. It seemed a reasonable question.

'Please lie quiet,' he said. 'You close you eyes.'

I responded like a good patient should. The prodding continued and then I heard, and felt, a sort of squelching, which made me open my eyes again, a little horrified. Had he broken the skin? What was he doing down there, disembowelling me? At one stage the pushing and prodding felt like some wild animal was trying to claw its way into me. He pushed, then eased off, then massaged the area firmly and pushed again; the expectation was that he would break through to get out whatever it was he was trying to get out. But this was just the expectation, I guess, because it never actually felt like the skin was broken. Despite this, I glanced up to see him whisking something away, something awful that he dropped in the bucket with a plop. I was too shocked to say anything, and no sooner had he done that than he had grabbed a cotton wool swab, dabbed some blood off my tummy — *my blood?* — and wiped it clean. I put my hand on the area he'd been working on and the skin was smooth and unbroken. There wasn't a mark on me. Even more miraculously, there wasn't a mark on his pristine white long sleeve Filipino shirt. The cotton wool swab, on the other hand, seemed soaked in blood. A neat trick.

'What the hell was that stuff?' I asked.

'It is no good,' he said. Not very specific but I got the picture.

Now I had seen this sort of thing on TV, and heard that they reputedly used pigs' blood and animal entrails hidden in their shirtsleeves, but I couldn't for the life of me work out how Felipe Cruz had managed to conceal these gizzards in this spartan room. His shirt was one of those see-through numbers, so there couldn't be anything concealed there. Before I had time to quiz him about what was going on, he told me to close my eyes again and he went back 'in'. I lay back and sort of moaned a bit as he prodded on.

A minute or so later I felt and heard the squelching again, and looked up to see something else messy apparently being retrieved from my lower abdomen. It looked like the mullet gut I used to use as bait when I was a keen fisherman in my teens. Had he got that from me? I had hardly felt a thing this time, just the slightest pressure as he pushed down on my tummy again. Meanwhile, he slung another bloody mess into the bucket, grabbed a new cotton wool swab and cleaned up. He worked quickly, like an expert chef over his stove, and again his shirt remained spotless. I looked at the sleeves, trying to suss if there were bulges in them where he had packets of chicken giblets sluicing around, but couldn't detect anything. His sleight-of-hand was amazing and he seemed fired up now, and went in again and again until, after about six goes, he declared that he had got it all. Despite being very squeamish, I wanted to have a look in the bucket to see what had been liberated from my person. Was I half the man I used to be? But he rang a small bell on his implement table and the maid came in, rather quickly I thought, and whisked the bucket away.

'That is all,' he declared. So I got up and put on my shirt and shoes again. The experience had been short and intense and I did feel a strange sort of relief – just some sort of placebo reaction, I imagined. How the hell had he done what he'd just done, I wondered?

The maid led me into the living room. I was to have a chat with Felipe and his wife during his break. Mary had enthusiastically promised them I would do a story on them, so I'd brought along a notebook just for show – I wasn't sure I really wanted to write anything. It all seemed too weird, really. Mary had, meanwhile, turned up and was sitting in the lounge room with the healer's wife, Maria. There was definitely some sort of hair thing going on in this family because Maria also had an amazingly thick head of dark black hair, sans the Brylcreem. She was dressed in black and wore a large gold cross on a chain around her neck and looked a bit Spanish, obviously having lineage from the Philippines' colonial era. She had a widow's peak like Eddie Munster's and the dress sense of Morticia Adams. We chatted over tea and Filipino sponge cake. I wondered where Felipe was but when I sat down I saw him outside at the edge of the canal and he appeared to be – this was strange – fishing. I couldn't quite believe my eyes at first.

'Is Felipe fishing out there?' I asked his wife.

'Oh yes,' said Maria. 'He like to relax between patients. He caught a pish lass week and want to catch one every day now.'

Those Gold Coast canals, which connect to the Nerang River, have more fish in them than you'd imagine, not to mention the odd shark. Fishing was a common pastime among people who lived on the canals, but it was a little surprising that Felipe was doing his fishing between patients. I mean, how many surgeons interrupt their operations so they can wet a line? The fact that he had a waiting room full of desperados didn't seem to bother him or his wife. How he could stand out there fishing while all those people sat inside waiting for him was beyond me. We sipped tea and chatted while he re-baited his hook and cast out again. Eventually he put the rod handle into a holder of some sort, leaving the line out, and came back inside. 'No pish today,' he said, and I wondered whether he had a pocket full of bait ready for his next session.

'You feeling better?' he asked me.

'Oh, yes, much better,' I said, because I thought I should.

'Isn't what Felipe does amazing?' said Mary.

'Oh, yes, amazing,' I said, looking round the spacious living room.

Though the house was sparsely decorated, everything was top of the range. There was obviously money in this faith-healing business and by now I was certain that was the point. Faith was one thing, but ripping people off was another, and by now my curiosity had turned to mild disgust. I wasn't sure how he achieved the illusion of his psychic surgery but I could see it was a cynical sham by a bloke who seemed more interested in angling than healing.

When I went to see Mary a couple of weeks later, I was pleased to hear she had gone off her Filipino faith-healing kick. She was now looking for a new guru.

'Any guru will do,' Bob commented.

'Maybe you should just find yourself a good yogi,' I suggested, trying to be helpful.

Bob started plucking at his guitar and said: 'Yeah . . . Yogi Bear.'

Walk like an Egyptian

'Do you happen to know who you were?' a small, birdlike woman asked, sidling up to me.

'I'm sorry?'

'Do you know who you were in your previous incarnations?' she asked again, very politely.

'I'm still trying to work out who the hell I am in this one,' I said.

'Ah, but it is important to know,' she insisted. 'There may be problems in this life that relate to unresolved issues in past lives. It's often the way.'

Issues. Oh yeah, I had plenty of issues.

'So if I was Lady Godiva or Josef Stalin or Arthur Caldwell, I should know about it for my own good?'

'Indeed,' she said. 'Have any of them come up?'

'Well, no, but I haven't really looked into it,' I said. 'We're just here to do a story today, actually. So with that in mind . . . can I ask how you came to find out about this — place?'

'Oh, we were guided here,' she said, and her husband, equally birdlike but slightly less wizened, nodded agreeably. 'The spirits led us. We feel we knew Cheryl and Dennis in former lives in ancient Egypt.'

'So you were ancient Egyptians in a previous incarnation too?' I asked.

'Oh yes, I think we all were really,' she said. 'It all comes from there, you know, all religion and spirituality emanates from that marvellous place and time. Harold and I were attendants in Pharaoh's court in those days. We have found that out since coming here but we felt we had been there even before verifying it with Dennis and Cheryl. When we first experienced this music, for example, we just knew we had heard it before.'

The music was certainly ethereal: it featured harp and oboe, which lent it an other-worldly sound.

'Déjà vu, all over again?' I suggested.

'Exactly,' she said, stuffing a small, crustless, salmon sandwich into her mouth.

We were in a pole house on the side of a hill in Kooralbyn Valley, a rural resort settlement in the countryside of southern Queensland, attending a seminar at the Meditational Arts, an organisation dedicated to the revival of a 3500-year-old ancient Egyptian tradition of music, dance and spirituality. But while it might have been just a pole house to Ripley — the photographer I worked with — and me, it was the equivalent of an Egyptian temple to everyone else. But it was a bloody long way from Karnak.

The high priestess here was Cheryl Stoll, and the head

priest her much older husband Dennis, an esteemed English conductor who had worked with Sir Thomas Beecham, a musical great who had spiritualist leanings and apparently believed he had been an ancient Egyptian in an earlier life – a court artist by the name of Khabekhnet, to be precise. Dennis and Cheryl, who was from the West Indies and looked like a Nubian queen dressed in her Egyptian clobber, had been reviving and promulgating ancient Egyptian music and wisdom in the UK for some years, but had moved camp to Australia looking for new acolytes; some might say 'suckers'. They'd obviously found some.

I'd found out about them when I saw a brochure advertising their meditation and seminar program at a natural therapies clinic I went to for shiatsu massage and acupuncture. The ancient Egyptian stuff intrigued me, and most people seem to have a penchant for it, so I figured it would make a good story for the rags I was writing for then, the sort of publications that used to be prescribed reading in barbershops. I specialised in weird and wonderful people stories, and there were quite a few of them on the Gold Coast.

I had an editor interested in this ancient Egyptian bizzo. 'Only in Queensland,' he'd said, so off I went to Kooralbyn for the day with Ripley, a bloke who couldn't be less interested in matters pertaining to his immortal soul. It was the weekend and the place was more than an hour's drive away, so he wasn't that keen until we got there and he learnt the seminar included some ancient Egyptian temple dancing by several nubile young women. These were sort of like the vestal virgins, I figured.

We spent a half-hour or so watching (I watched, Ripley gawked) the temple dancing – which consisted of a lot of gliding around in fancy dress – accompanied by music Dennis had composed. He was convinced he was the reincarnation of an ancient Egyptian temple music composer and had formed his own group – the Nefer Ensemble – back in London to re-imagine the lost music of Egyptian antiquity. It was pretty divine stuff actually, and what with the music, the costumes and the girls wafting around the room, it was pretty heady. Weird but heady.

After the dancing and a bit of a talk about how wonderful the ancient kingdom by the Nile was, we had our lunchbreak, which was a chance for some chit-chat with the folks who had forked out hard cash for their trip down a 3500-year-old memory lane. 'Fruitcakes' was a word which came to mind after a few conversations over the sandwich table.

After the lunchbreak the seminar continued with a session on the Sacred Way of Star Wisdom, which was Cheryl's speciality.

'The rediscovery of the Star Wisdom is the most important breakthrough in our comprehension of ancient Egypt since Champollion deciphered the Rosetta Stone,' explained Dennis, introducing the session. 'The ability to read the divine destiny of an individual at birth, to foresee natural disasters such as flood and famine, and to help humanity to live in accord with the 42 cosmic laws, instead of fighting against them, is one which the sages of this ancient civilisation possessed to a high degree. The 42 divine laws control the visible and invisible worlds. These are changeless as the tides, constant as the movements of the planets and the stars.'

'If you say so, sport,' said Ripley out of the side of his mouth.

Cheryl then gave her little talk on the ancient Star Wisdom, and during it I noticed that Ripley had started looking at his watch intermittently. The ancient Egyptian temple dancing was done with, and without that Ripley's interest was waning fast.

'Look, I've got to have another quick chat with them at the afternoon tea break, then we'll head off,' I said, trying to placate him. I could see he was hoping that if we took off now he might catch the tail-end of the annual Gold Coast media piss-up he was missing. By the time I was finally ready to leave, Ripley's mood had turned positively sour and he was already in the car revving the engine when Cheryl came out to wave us off. I wondered what the neighbours thought of these comings and goings and folk walking around dressed like ancient Egyptians. They probably thought Cheryl got about in her nightie all day.

The Stolls were fascinating people, whether you believed what they were on about or not. Dennis was obviously a man of great accomplishments, who had rubbed shoulders with the great and the good in his life as a composer and conductor. He had even been friendly with the famous spiritual teacher Krishnamurti for a time. Cheryl meanwhile was passionate about what she was doing and had apparently received a visitation from the Virgin Mary during a bout of fever when she was a little girl in Jamaica. The Holy

Mother had told her she had spiritual gifts which she would share with the world. Some might have interpreted that as a call to enter a nunnery, but Cheryl's mission turned out to be rather different.

It did seem weird that she and Dennis were doing their eternal work at Kooralbyn, which is in the middle of nowhere globally speaking, but then again its ancient equivalents produced similarly anomalous flowerings. I mean, Nazareth was supposed to be a dead-end town where nothing ever happened, wasn't it?

'Nutters,' was Ripley's frank assessment as we drove out of the lost valley.

'Yeah, nutters,' I agreed. But the problem was that I seemed to be innately attracted to nutters at that time. I mean the whole thing seemed highly unlikely but my imagination had been tickled. There was something enchanting about the idea, and sometimes we all hanker for the good old days – and they don't get much older than 1500 BC.

I didn't mention to Ripley that Cheryl had invited me to come back and spend a weekend at the pole house temple getting my star chart done, learning more about the 42 divine laws of Star Wisdom – which seemed like rather a lot – and having some healing massages. Healing massages? I liked the sound of that and went back, by myself this time, a few weeks later.

I was living at home with my mum and brother at the time. My brother didn't seem very surprised by anything I got up to, and Mum just sort of rolled her eyes when I told her I was heading back to Kooralbyn for the weekend.

'How much will it cost?' she asked, suspecting a rip-off.

'It's by special invitation because I've done a story on them,' I explained. 'It won't cost me a shekel.'

So I pointed my trusty Holden Gemini in the direction of ancient Egypt, via Kooralbyn Valley. The Stolls had arranged accommodation for me at the Kooralbyn Valley Resort, which is where their guests stayed and, more enticingly, where the dancers were living. It was a mixture of residential and resort, with the emphasis on recreation. Lots of golfers and horsey people wandered around dressed for the part and looking rather pleased with themselves.

The morning after I arrived I had a massage from Cheryl, followed by a reading of my star chart with a view to working out which of the 42 cosmic laws I needed to bone up on. Apparently each month had a theme in this Star Wisdom business. January's was discipline, February's holy breath, March was innocence, and April, wisdom – you get the picture. And each month had divine laws attached to it – things like... listen to the small voice within... surrender to God... the eternal moment is now... we all come from the light... we are members of one another – the sort of thing you might read on the back bumper-bar of any Kombi van heading for Nimbin.

My previous incarnations were delved into, too, though they appeared a bit murky. At least I had not been a mass murderer or anything awful – in ancient Egypt I was apparently some sort of second-string priest, which seemed exotic enough if a little disappointing. But thankfully I wasn't one of those poor bastards who had to lug those bloody great

Any Guru Will Do

stone blocks across the sand to make the pyramids. Nobody ever seems to have been a shit-kicker when they delve into your past lives, though, do they? If you're not a king or queen, you're always something interesting. You'll never hear people who are reincarnations of ancient Egyptians telling you that they shovelled camel dung for a living back in the days of the pharaohs.

'I can see you grieving over the loss of someone close, an unexpected loss,' Cheryl said, closing her eyes. 'After this loss you dedicate yourself to temple life. Aeons from then I can see an Oriental setting.'

'A Chinese restaurant?'

'It's a courtly setting,' she said. 'You were . . . some sort of Mandarin.'

'Oh,' I said. 'That sounds nice. As long as I wasn't Genghis Khan.'

'No,' she said quite seriously. 'But I've met someone who was.'

I *think* she was kidding.

After my private session I joined a group in the living room – or 'inner sanctum', as they liked to call it – for a talk by Dennis about the music and dance of ancient Egypt.

'The music of this time is a pure source of modal music,' he explained. 'It reflected their philosophy of love. The ancient Egyptians spoke of the intelligence of the heart. Their art and music was the product of love.'

Ancient Egypt was obviously a wonderful place where they all danced and sang and praised the high heavens. Being Pharaoh would have been alright, I suppose – being carried around in a chair fanned with palm fronds all day. Mind you, it must have been pretty tough for everyone beneath the aristocracy. It couldn't have been such a great place for Moses and his mob, for instance, because they sure got the hell out of there as soon as they could. But then, they had a little help.

But the idea of having lived before didn't seem that outrageous. Many of us have felt unusual kinships with cultures or places of the ancient world, and it's rather fun to imagine having been some kind of potentate in the ancient world. There is also something terribly attractive about ancient Egypt, or the idea of it at least. The articles and documentaries about it just keep on coming, and the sense of magic it conjures must make even non-believers think again, if only for a brief, flickering moment.

But all that was, as they say in the classics, a long, long time ago. I visited the Meditational Arts a couple more times in the vain hope that one of the temple dancers might take a shine to me, but with Cheryl acting as den mother that was never on the cards – or should I say in the cards.

Then I found some other New Age distraction, lost touch with the joint and never heard anything of the Stolls again until recently, when I ran into a friend, Carol, who had kept in touch with Cheryl over the years.

Dennis had gone to his reward, she told me, and was obviously up yonder with the Shining Ones, the ancient Egyptian equivalent of the angels. Cheryl was now living in New York, painting and still involved in dance.

'So she's still doing that ancient Egyptian folk dancing?'

'No, she's into Latin dance now,' Carol said.

'Latin? You're kidding.' I was gobsmacked. I just couldn't see the connection. That blew my recollections of Cheryl serenely padding around the temple at Kooralbyn right out of the water.

'What about ancient Egypt? What about the sacred temple music? What about the Shining Ones?'

'Their time is done, for now,' Carol said.

Had Cheryl discovered that she'd been a famous Brazilian dancer in her most immediate past life and decided to use her recollections to get a bit more rhythm in her life? I'll never know...

'Crikey, the dogs bark, the caravan moves on,' I said, somewhat crestfallen. I mean, for a couple of decades I'd had this idyllic image in my mind of Cheryl and her temple dancers floating around in their mock-chiffon gowns like angels come to earth. What was I left with now? An image of an aged Cheryl in a lamé bikini samba-ing her way through the evenings in the Big Apple, tangoing with some Latin lothario. Oh, it was too cruel, far too cruel, and I told Carol as much.

'People change from life to life,' she said.

'Yeah,' I shrugged. 'I guess a girl's got... to make a living.'

Dr Wong, I Presume?

'Make it look like a monkey,' said Dr Wong as he clenched his teeth and sneered at me. 'Like diss.'

'Okay,' I said, baring my teeth, stretching my face and straining every tendon in my neck.

'Dat is good, dat is good . . . now hold one moment, relax and repeat.'

I contorted my face again and again following his instructions.

'Dat is da face exercise,' he said, stating the bleeding obvious. 'Velly good for you.'

'As long as no-one sees you doing it,' I said.

'Is not matter what people think,' he said. 'But you can do in private, anyhow. So dat is okay.'

'Sure,' I said.

'Now I show you some tai chi.'

This was my first consultation with Dr Cyril Wong. It was actually the first time I had ever consulted somebody who practised Chinese medicine, even though I'd spent most of my childhood in Hong Kong. It was a British colony back then, and Europeans tended to see European doctors, of course. We knew there was a whole other world of what seemed like Chinese hocus-pocus to us, and we knew that it involved weird medicines which were very different to what we took. I was fascinated by the Chinese apothecaries I used to see around Kowloon, though I'd hold my nose when I passed them. All those dried bits and pieces displayed in bins out front stank to high heaven as far as I was concerned. There were antlers and all sorts of other weird-looking roadkill in the windows – some things that looked like desiccated dog turds or bits of monkey's entrails. My amah would occasionally stink out the kitchen late at night preparing a witch's brew made of this stuff. But I'd never tried the local ways when it came to health. Now, decades later, here I was giving it a whirl with Dr Wong.

'You know tai chi?' Dr Wong asked.

'No, but I know his brother, lychee,' I said, but that didn't seem to register. 'I do, of course. Actually, when I was a boy in Hong Kong I used to see people doing tai chi all the time.'

That was in the 1960s, well before the tai chi craze hit Australia. In Kowloon Tong, where we lived, the parks were full of people dancing in slow motion, particularly in the early morning. My neighbourhood pals and I were always amazed by their concentration and would often taunt them, pulling faces, running around in front of them, trying to see if we could disturb them – but we were rarely successful. Now I was learning some of the rudimentary moves, finally.

'Now you try dis,' said Dr Wong, standing with his legs slightly apart and pushing down with his palms. 'Dat is da Qigong, more powerful than tai chi. Maybe you can learn sometime? All will help energy.'

This first session felt like the Idiot's Express Guide to Oriental Medicine, starting and finishing with advanced face-pulling. But I was desperate, so if my wellbeing depended on trying to look like a monkey, I was prepared to give it a go. I had been suffering for months from migraines and a general feeling of malaise, which in retrospect seems almost certain to have had something – or perhaps everything – to do with the fact that I was working at the time for Brisbane City Council. Between jobs in journalism, I'd got a gig in the council's Information Services section, a department dedicated to stopping any information getting out. I wasn't used to working in a huge bureaucracy where life was an endless round of meetings at which nothing was ever decided. Nor was I used to the comparatively early starts, so I was always late for work. This had annoyed a couple of my colleagues, who had dobbed me in to the boss of the department, a very genial bloke by the name of Brian Grace. He had reluctantly hauled me into his office on the matter.

'Phil, I hate to have to do this, but unfortunately I have to respond when I get a complaint,' he said.

'Fair enough,' I said.

'Now you know that we work on flexitime and that the latest possible time you can start in the morning is 8.45?'

'Is it?'

'Yes it is. So in future do you think you could possibly get here by then?'

'Well, Brian, I can try but I can't guarantee anything.'

He shrugged his shoulders and I went back to my desk. The fact is that with things like that going on and the endless drudgery of the work, I was, as they say, 'internalising'. Consequently, I felt nauseous at work and had migraines every couple of weeks. I spent a lot of time in the surgery of the very nice GP whose rooms were at the top of the office tower I worked in. They had their own doctor up there, I imagine, because working at the council obviously made a lot of people sick. I would be in the doctor's office eyrie at least once a week having my heart listened to, my blood pressure taken, my reflexes checked. Blood tests were run, too, but she couldn't find anything wrong with me.

'Perhaps you might find some form of natural therapy more helpful,' she'd said one day in an obvious gambit to get rid of me. I mean, since when do medicos recommend the opposition? 'The only other option is some sort of medication, and I'd rather not go down that route if we can help it,' she continued. 'There's a Chinese fellow in Fortitude Valley who I've heard is very good. Do you think you'd like to try that?'

'I'll try anything once,' I said, 'sometimes twice.'

So I had made an appointment to see a certain Dr Wong during my lunch hour a few days later. His rooms were in a former light industrial building down a side street and there was a mild, slightly bitter herbal smell in the air as

I entered. There was no-one on the reception desk when I arrived so I rang the small bell on the counter.

'Yes, hello,' said a Chinese man who came out of the room behind.

'Dr Wong, I presume?'

'Yes, of course,' he said. 'May you come in?'

The consultation began with a checking of my pulse, which was declared to be rather disappointing. 'Diss pulse is weak,' he said. 'Too yin. Have to make some yang to balance.'

He felt my head. 'There is imbalance in the body. Too much cold. If too much cold, must make it hot; if too much heat, must make it cold.'

'That makes sense,' I said.

'You see there,' he said pointing to the wall. There was a chart of the various sorts of chi ... wind, heat, cold, damp, dryness and summer wind. 'Dere must be balance of element. If no balance, big problem.'

'I understand,' I said.

'You understand here,' he said, pointing to my head. 'But you muss understand in here and here and here.' He touched his chest, heart and stomach. I nodded.

'Do you sleep?'

'I sleep okay, most of the time.'

'Do you get the headache?'

'Oh yes, I get the headache alright.'

'Do you ejacurrate too much?'

'Pardon?' I wasn't sure if I'd heard right.

'Ejacurrate,' he said.

'Do I?'

'Yes, do you ejacurrate?'

'Well I certainly hope so.'

'Maybe you ejacurrate too much. This may weaken the system. Too much ejacurration can make da vessel empty. You must keep the vessel from being too empty.'

'I see,' I said.

'So not too much ejacurration.'

I felt like I had walked into the middle of a Benny Hill sketch, or a Woody Allen movie. What was that line of Woody's again about masturbation? 'Don't knock it . . . it's sex with someone I love.'

'I'll keep that in mind,' I said, keen to move on.

Then he took me through some exercise routines, and we were just finishing them when a woman popped her head around the corner. 'Next patient here,' she said – quite rudely, I thought.

'Okay, okay,' Dr Wong said, adding with what seemed like some aggravation: 'Dat is my wife.' He scribbled some Chinese characters on a piece of note paper. 'You give this to her for medicine and come back next week,' he said.

Outside, Mrs Wong measured out some pellets of what looked like animal droppings into a small plastic bottle and scribbled on the label. 'You muss take three tablet each day,' she barked. 'Do not forget.'

I nodded meekly. This seemed straightforward enough, although I can't say there was much effect. I was expecting some magical reaction from these mystical Chinese herb balls but nothing much seemed to happen after taking them for a few days.

I did the facial exercises, too, in the bathroom with the door closed so my girlfriend, Sandra, didn't have to witness them, and made a half-hearted stab at the rudimentary Qigong movements. That didn't last long, though, because he'd said to do them in the morning and mornings are not my best time. The most I can manage at that time of the day is the lifting of a cup of tea.

Meanwhile, work at the council was as enervating as usual and I went back to Dr Wong week after week. He soon decided acupuncture might be the best approach and turned me into a human pin-cushion in a side room while he attended to other patients, occasionally coming in to tweak the needles like some torturer. The acupuncture made me feel a bit better, actually. Even Western doctors seemed to approve of it, to a degree at least, and what the Chinese do with acupuncture is amazing. I had seen a documentary where they operated on people using acupuncture. The patients were lying there with their eyes open while the surgeons messed around with their gizzards. Not my idea of fun, but impressive.

After one session Dr Wong took my pulse again. 'Still cold,' he said. 'Too cold mean poor circulation, digestion no good. Still need a lot of work.'

'I'm feeling a bit fluey too at the moment,' I said.

'Yes, because system not working, immunity can be low. Too much phlegm. I think, maybe you need some strong Chinese medicine, make it clear out. Have you ever mix up da Chinese herb to take?'

'Only those pills you gave me.'

'No no, dat is not strong enough,' he said. 'You must get da real herb and make it up yourself. Make it like soup to drink.'

'Oh yes,' I said. 'I know what you mean but I've never tried that.'

'Okay, I give,' he said writing some Chinese characters on a prescription pad, tearing off a piece of paper and handing it to me.

'You can go Chinatown, get diss and make a soup for drink,' he said. So when I left I went straight to a Chinese store I knew. I sometimes bought tea and Chinese sausages and other provisions there. This time I went to the counter where all the Chinese herbs were dished out and handed the guy behind the counter my slip of paper. He examined it for a minute trying to make out the prescription. It seems to be a universal problem that chemists can't make out doctors' handwriting.

Once he'd worked out what was on the script, he brightened and started enthusiastically scooping stuff from various little bins he had behind the counter. He put the gunk — which looked like sticks, bark and dried leaves — into small, brown paper bags and wrote something on the outside of each one, but since it was in Chinese I had no idea what it said. Then, when he'd finished making up about five bags of the gear, he put them all into a larger plastic bag and then handed me a little piece of paper with some simple instructions written in English on how to prepare the stuff.

'You can read?' he said.

'Yes I can,' I said.

'You can make it like soup,' he said.

'Yes I can,' I repeated. I took the bag back to work with me and kept it under my desk.

The smell wafted around the office a bit and I was getting a few funny looks by the end of the afternoon.

'Chinese herbs,' I explained when the boss went by, sniffing.

'As long as you don't smoke them in here,' he said.

'They're for drinking, not smoking,' I said. He looked suspicious.

I put them in the kitchen that evening and was filling a saucepan with water when Sandra came home.

'You're not going to do that now, are you?' she said.

'Well, I thought I might,' I said. 'I feel dreadful.'

'You'll probably feel even worse after you take all that stuff,' she said, looking into the bowl I had mixed the dried ingredients in.

'It's supposed to make me feel better.'

'Yes, but I think you should take it in the morning rather than at night. You won't be able to sleep properly with all that sloshing around inside.'

So I agreed to leave it until the next day, particularly since Friday night was pizza night, a ritual. After the pizza we each ate a huge bowl of ice cream. This was done usually watching a B-grade movie.

The next day we were due to go to a wedding in the afternoon, something I'd temporarily forgotten. So I thought I'd better take my herbs around mid-morning, well before we had to get ready to go out. I boiled some water, emptied the herbs into it and watched it start bubbling.

'Double, double toil and trouble; fire burn and cauldron bubble,' I was chanting as Sandra came in.

'What died in here?' she said. 'That smells absolutely foul.'

'Diss make it hot if cold, make it cold if hot,' I said, impersonating Dr Wong. 'Diss make my chi flow, balance out my yin and yang.'

'That will probably blow your yin right out the other side of your yang,' she said.

'No way,' I said. 'The Chinese have been taking this stuff for thousands of years.'

'It smells like it,' Sandra said.

'Soup of the gods,' I said, stirring it some more.

Following the instructions, I boiled the stuff for a little while longer and then strained it into a small glass jug. I got a soup cup and went outside and poured myself a cup and started slowly sipping at it.

'Jesus,' I said. 'This is pretty rough stuff. But I guess it's a case of no pain, no gain.'

The thickish black goop was bitter as hell, and each time I swallowed a mouthful I shivered uncontrollably for a few seconds. But I was determined to finish it. I mean, the Chinese were knocking back this stuff and healing themselves with acupuncture when we were still scratching our names on the ground with sticks, so they should know what they're doing. Right?

'Confucius say, man who drink Chinese herb medicine soup in morning is new man by afternoon,' I said.

'Yes, well, Confucius better be right because we've got a wedding to go to, don't forget.'

My friend, Ian Spence, was marrying his fiancée, Madonna, that afternoon at a garden ceremony in Brisbane's leafy west. As we drove out to the place, I was feeling as well as could be expected for someone who never really felt that well.

It was a lovely service in the green setting, and afterwards we all repaired to the function centre attached for the reception. We had eaten dinner and the speeches were under way when I started to feel a bit odd. I checked the pulse in my neck to see if it was racing — it was. It felt like jungle drums beating away just under the skin.

'What's the matter with you?' asked Sandra.

'I don't know,' I said. 'I feel a bit squiffy.'

'Well, is that something new?'

'I guess not.' I felt decidedly odd, and then I started to feel clammy. My palms were sweating, so I dried them on my napkin and loosened my tie.

'You're alright,' Sandra said.

'Easy for you to say,' I said.

And that was when the Chinese herbs finally made their move. All of a sudden it felt like the entire contents of my stomach were being drained. There was a gurgling like a gushing creek in my belly and what sounded like a toilet flushing in my abdomen. It was loud enough for those seated near me to hear — a couple of people looked around.

'What the hell was that?' Sandra asked.

'Um, I think the Chinese herbs are on the march.'

'Oh, great. I mean, did you have to take them today?'

'Well, you said not to take them last night,' I whinged. Meanwhile the flushing continued until there was a last trickling gurgle.

'Oh, God,' I said, getting up.

'Where are you going?' Sandra asked.

'Where do you think?' I pushed my chair out from the table, got up and rushed from the room, much to the surprise of the other guests, who must have wondered what was up. I went back out into the foyer desperately looking for the loo. Soon I found a door with a symbol of a man in a top hat on it. When was the last time you ran into anyone wearing a top hat to the dunny? I thought as I burst in the door and rushed to the cubicle. I was in there for at least half an hour. The Chinese herbs were, to say the least, purgative. They seemed to have worked like a time bomb, sitting latent in my gut for hours before finally exploding. By the time I got back to the table dessert had been served.

'You're as white as a sheet,' said Sandra.

'I know,' I said. 'I'm half the man I used to be. Bugger Dr Wong.'

But I went back to see him the following week, a few kilos lighter.

'You looking much better,' he said. 'Chinese medicine work, yes?'

'It certainly had some effect,' I said. 'But I think I lost a few vital internal organs along the way.'

'Huh?'

'I mean, no, I guess it must have done something. I don't feel like I have a flu coming on any more.' No flu could survive that stuff, I thought.

Back at work, things went from bad to worse. In my cubicle at Information Services each hour felt like a day, each day like a week – and no amount of acupuncture or Chinese herbs could change that. I decided my detour into the public sector was a mistake I had to rectify, even though Dr Wong had suggested prudence in the face of unemployment.

'Chinese have old saying,' he said. ' "Keep riding donkey until horse come along".'

'But what if you fall off the donkey and it starts kicking you in the head?'

'Find horse fast,' he said.

Despite that inscrutable Oriental wisdom, I resigned a few weeks later. I recall almost floating down the Queen Street Mall after leaving that office forever. And in no time I was feeling fine, which was no surprise to Sandra, who reckoned my symptoms were psychosomatic anyway. I went back to see Dr Wong only once after that and I told him I had quit.

'What you do now?' he asked.

'Just see what turns up,' I said. 'We're thinking of going overseas for a holiday first, though.'

'Journey of thousand mile begin with first step,' he said. 'Now let me feel you pulse again.'

At Last, a Cure!

I sat in the naturopath's waiting room reading about how wheatgrass can save the world. You never read this sort of stuff in doctors' surgeries, do you? It's all *Woman's Day* and *New Idea*. Here there were ads for portable pyramids and Tantric yoga, and pictures of impossibly healthy people – unlike the naturopath himself, who turned out to be a long, tall streak of misery. But he had something of a reputation and I was desperate to find someone who might cure my mystery illness.

I was willing to try anything because I had been crook since our honeymoon in Malaysia some months earlier. Sandra and I had spent most of the happy occasion on Tioman Island, a jungly jewel in the South China Sea. It had been an exotic and memorable trip, but for me the memory was lingering much longer than it should after a bad case of food poisoning on the island. (I got sunstroke and seasickness too, but that's another story.) It was, we figured, something in the noodles, and the after-effects were still with me when we arrived back in Brisbane. And not long after we got home from Tioman we had a major upheaval in our life – we moved to Melbourne, where Sandra had been offered a job as a writer on *TV Week* magazine. I was, meanwhile, left to scratch together a living, which included some casual reporting shifts at *The Sunday Age*, where they seemed amazed that I could even use a computer, let alone write. They had funny ideas about people from Queensland – thought we communicated through grunts and whistles.

Getting married, moving cities, trying to scrounge a living – the stress of it all was exacerbated by the lingering, mysterious affliction I had carried back from Tioman. For months I'd been waking in the middle of the night shaking and sweating, mopping my brow with the sheets and exhorting Sandra to call an ambulance or, on one occasion, even a priest. I was convinced it was something serious – maybe malaria or some exotic disease modern man had forgotten but which lingered in the steamy, primeval jungles waiting to pounce on the poor unsuspecting tourist. Sandra reckoned it was just a tummy bug.

Whatever it was, it seemed to be undetectable to modern medicine, which had prodded and probed me to no avail back in Brissie. I had exhausted orthodox opinion, which had found nothing despite an exhaustive series of blood tests and other probings. I was a virtual pin-cushion at the end of that process and could easily have been mistaken for a junkie by the tracks on my arms. I was given a course of strong antibiotics and told to drink lots of water.

But during our first few weeks in Melbourne I was still ill. I would sit bolt upright in bed each night, usually around 1 a.m., shivering and shaking and calling out to God. Sandra had taken to sleeping through all this, and so my regular pleas for an ambulance went unheeded. I wandered the house trussed up in my gown looking like the ghost of Christmas past. There wasn't much room to wander, though, because the joint we lived in – an attractive Victorian terrace house in trendy Albert Park – was about the size of a postage stamp and had little in it besides some kitchen stuff, a desk, some large cushions serving in lieu of a couch, and the futon we slept on, which I was finding harder and harder to raise myself from each morning.

After a month of this, a Melbourne friend suggested I see her naturopath, a guy called Jerry. He had apparently cured her of a variety of ailments. He was at Frankston, a singly unattractive place about a half-hour away along Port Phillip Bay. I had made the trek there in good faith and after 15 minutes he deigned to see me. I thought he had another patient who had been holding him up but I think he was actually just having his morning tea.

'What are your symptoms?' he asked, after I was ushered into a small, spartan room with a poster of a dolphin on the wall behind his desk.

'Nausea, night sweats, shivering, temperatures and a feeling of imminent death.'

He nodded and produced a stethoscope. 'Hmm, there's a slight murmur in the heart,' he said, applying the cold bit between my upper shirt buttons. 'And your chi seems to be quite severely blocked.'

'What causes that?'

'Depletion and enervation,' he offered. It was a diagnosis I could probably have made myself. He asked me to poke out my tongue and then peered into my eyes. 'The digestive tract is quite upset,' he said, getting up and moving a small electrical-looking unit on wheels over beside me. Then he handed me two metallic tubes with wires attached that led back into the housing of the machine. It looked like something out of *The Ipcress File* and I thought, the bastard's going to torture a diagnosis out of me!

'Hold on to those tightly,' he said, gesturing towards the tubes, which I was handling like two sticks of gelignite.

'What are they for?'

'They will measure your energy levels and give me an accurate reading of the mean age of your body,' he said. 'We all age at different rates and the physiological age can often be different from your actual age. So your external age and internal age may differ quite considerably.'

'Really?' I said. What the hell was he talking about?

'Yes,' he said, fiddling with the wires like some nutty professor. 'In fact the internal body age is like a clock, to a certain extent. By visualisation and correct living you can change that mean age. You can actually set your body clock to the age you aspire to be. It's a technique yogis have been using for thousands of years. I have set mine for my mid-twenties.'

That being the case, I wanted to ask why he looked like a wasted, middle-aged hippie.

Meanwhile I kept gripping the shiny metal tubes in my clammy paws, hoping not to be zapped in the process. I didn't want to go home with an Afro. The naturopath, Jerry, monitored a needle that was wavering back and forth on a small screen on top of the unit, which looked to me awfully like a Geiger counter.

'So what do you think?' I asked. 'What's my half-life?'

'Well, it's rather alarming,' he said.

'How alarming?'

'Well, according to this, your actual bodily age is 63,' he said with a sense of certainty mixed with foreboding and accentuated by a shaking of the head – the sort of head-shaking you get from a second-hand car dealer when they lift the bonnet of your car. Considering I was only 36 at the time, this was rather bad news.

'Sixty-three!' I said. 'Crikey, I don't feel a day over 61.'

He remained taciturn and started jotting things on my patient card with some urgency. When he'd examined the reading from the machine again, as if he doubted the evidence, he turned back to me.

'What you're experiencing is related to a severe degradation of the integrity of your bodily systems due to the denuding of the reserves of a number of vital vitamins and minerals. All of this is exacerbated by an imbalance in your energy centres. Your chakras, that is.'

'Is it fixable?' I asked.

'With a rigorous program, over time.'

'How much time?'

'Oh, months... possibly years,' he smiled. I was

starting to twig to the way this guy did business. First the bad news – you were stuffed; then the good news – he could fix you. But that would take years, and how many thousands of dollars in consultations and treatments over that time? Meanwhile, he gave me a dietary sheet to follow that excluded almost everything, and some pamphlets. Then he loaded me up with a bag full of enough vitamins, minerals and homoeopathic remedies to treat a small country town and a graph that mapped out the quantities I was to take and the various times of day they should be self-administered. It looked like I would be a very busy boy. With all that in a paper bag, I paid up and left. I had dropped a couple of hundred bucks in the space of around 45 minutes.

'Do you really need all that stuff?' Sandra asked when she got home and saw the multitude of containers and bottles on the kitchen table.

'Since I apparently have the body of a 63-year-old, I guess I do.'

Even though I thought he was a nut, I'd pledged to follow the regimen he had set me – which just goes to show how desperate and confused I was. But by the time I was due to see him again a fortnight later, I was sick and tired of the whole routine – the tablets, the tinctures, the herbs, morning, noon and night – and since I wasn't feeling any better, I chucked the bloody lot. A terrible waste of money but quite liberating. I cancelled my next appointment and that was a relief, too. I mean, my bodily age had been 63 then so what might it be next time?

I didn't fancy being an octogenarian while still in my thirties.

In the meantime I'd met a guy who lived a few doors down and was into Transcendental Meditation. He suggested Ayurvedic medicine might help. They've been using it on the subcontinent for thousands of years, he told me. The subtext was that he thought if I visited the Maharishi Vedic Centre, the bearded one's HQ in Melbourne, I might also be brought into the fold. As an old Beatles fan from way back, the Maharishi was a familiar figure and TM sounded harmless enough, although all that levitating they claimed to do while meditating was a bit suss. But I was still ill and thought I'd try another tack. So I trotted off to see the Ayurvedic doctor at Maharishi central.

I expected some Indian guy in traditional clothing but he was Australian and he looked very much like a chartered accountant (in fact everyone at the centre looked like a chartered accountant). Ayurveda is based on treating bodily types known as the Tridoshas, which influence all movements, sensory functions and everything else of a bodily nature. The Tridoshas – basically, the three main bodily types – are Vata, Pitta and Kapha. After studying my pulse, which is apparently how they determine your body type, I was declared a Vata–Pitta hybrid, which was tantamount to a nervous wreck – not exactly news to me. This could all be helped, however, by meditation, which I promised to consider but had no intention of doing. I had, of course, tried meditation before – a couple of times, as it happens – but I think my experience with Dadaji all those years earlier had scarred me for life on that score. One never quite gets over being sprung, by a perfect stranger, dangling one's private parts in a basin. Whenever I tried to meditate I seemed to have flashbacks of that disturbing incident long ago.

I was given some rather lovely tea to drink to help calm me down – it had licorice, cardamom and all sorts of other yummy, spicy stuff in it, and was the only herbal tea I've ever drunk which I actually liked. I also bought, at the doctor's suggestion, a CD, which I was to play every night to heighten spiritual awareness. I played it as we were going to sleep the following few nights and it did calm me down – at least until I had my next turn.

The turns were not coming as often now but they were still upsetting. Sandra's theory was that whatever I'd picked up was slowly diminishing in power, which sounded fair enough. But I was sick of hovering on the verge of sleep wondering if I'd be jolted awake again with the heebie-jeebies in the middle of the night no matter how much Ayurvedic tea I drank.

By this stage daily life was becoming more stable since I was getting work in Melbourne and had shifted camp from the snooty Fairfax broadsheet to the Murdoch stable, where I got a job writing feature articles three days a week for *The Sunday Herald-Sun*, a good, honest tabloid where I felt more at home. I had also been hired to write a showbiz column for *Australasian Post* magazine. The editor at the time was a man with a very sick sense of humour. He insisted on calling the column 'The Dirt Pile with Filthy Phil' and I agreed for one very good reason. Money.

Each week I'd have to interview some local personality for my page – everyone from Maurie Fields to the Doug Anthony Allstars and even, once, Dame Edna Everage. She's a great bloke.

A few weeks into this gig I was interviewing a Melbourne comedian at his home in Elwood. This guy was making a comeback after being off the circuit for a while due to illness. He had regained his health after visiting a healer in nearby St Kilda.

'What sort of healer?' I asked.

'Hard to say what sort of healer he is,' he said, with a hint of mystery. 'All I know is that whatever he did worked.' The interview was pretty prosaic. Comedians are always so depressing. But I was interested – very interested – in his healer, still desperate for relief from the affliction which was intermittently ravaging me. I got a name and number for the healer before I left.

I was ambivalent at first about following up, though, because it might just be another dead-end, like so many others I had been driven to in my never-ending search for the magic bullet of health and wellbeing. I was starting to think it might actually be better to forget about searching for a cure and just put up with how I was — and save myself the angst of forever seeking completion. Because the problem was that whenever I tried to solve a problem, I usually found out that I was actually worse off than I thought. This couldn't be good for one's health, could it? But I couldn't help myself. Maybe I was actually an optimist? Because I always thought: maybe *this* time it would be the real deal.

That afternoon I rang to make an appointment with the apparently mystical Alan, who turned out to look anything but mystical when I turned up for my appointment with him a few days later. He lived in a tatty old terrace house in a rubbish-strewn side street in St Kilda. Alan was the size of your average garden gnome and his page-boy haircut made him vaguely resemble Davy Jones of the Monkees. But he seemed like a happy chappie, and he led me cheerfully down a dark, dank hallway — there were patches of mould along it — and into a rather spare kitchen, where he offered me the obligatory cup of herbal tea.

'I like to chat a bit before a treatment,' he said, gazing past me as he spoke. 'It gives me a general idea of which way to go, how to work with your particular energy field.'

'How exactly do you work?' I asked, sipping a cup of rose-hip tea. I hate rosehip tea.

'I work with the subtle body,' he explained, 'with the forces and energies that drive us, forces and energies that modern medicine knows nothing about. There are things happening in our minds and bodies which we aren't aware of most of the time but they are still having an effect.'

He still looked around me rather than at me, and I thought he must have been sizing up my aura. He asked me about my physical symptoms and my life in general, and after we had finished the tea he led me back down the hallway and into his sparsely furnished front room. There was just a desk, a chair and a massage table in there. On the walls were some framed photos of American Indian chiefs, their noble but rather sad visages staring out at me. Dangling from the window was one of those Native American dream-catcher things that you see in hippie shops. These little circles — with string tied across them to form a sort of web — and attendant feathers are based on real Native American charms, supposedly used to catch bad dreams before they arrive. Mind you, if I'd had one of them hanging above my bed when I was a kid, I would have been completely spooked. Alan's was, I presumed, to catch bad vibes on their way in from the ether. There were also a few other pictures of ethereal-looking beings — saints? angels? — propped on his desk. These were, Alan explained (because I asked), 'spirit guides'.

He hovered as I spread myself out on the massage table after following his instructions to take my shoes, socks, wedding ring and watch off. I waited for him to start doing whatever it was he did. I wasn't sure what to expect but was willing to give it a whirl because he seemed nice enough. He had a good vibe, as they say. Nothing seemed to be happening so I closed my eyes and waited. Then, after a few minutes, I opened them again to see Alan just standing there, hands outstretched, eyes shut, mumbling some sort of incantation. I thought I'd better shut my eyes again and let him get on with it.

Soon I began to hear a sort of whooshing noise above me. What is it with this whooshing sound anyway? I remember the same sort of sound being used to conjure up the Holy Spirit during my dalliance with born-again Christianity, but surely whatever Alan was conjuring up had nothing to do with that... Although I guess one shouldn't assume that the Holy Spirit is exclusively at the beck and call of the God-botherers. I peeked through half-closed lids to see him executing sweeping movements over me, like some kind of shaman – the type of thing you might see in a *National Geographic* special about witchdoctors in Borneo. But any decent witchdoctor would have a switch or something covered in feathers, which he could shake at you to exorcise the malady – wouldn't he? Alan was just using his hands, waving them slowly, then quickly, with the attendant whooshing. Whether this was having any effect on me or not was hard to gauge this early in the piece, but I certainly felt relaxed, lying prone on the massage table in the middle of the afternoon, enjoying my siesta.

Soon Alan turned on a sound system – a little player I hadn't noticed before. Chanting slowly filled the room, rising and falling to a background of soft but insistent drumming. Alan stopped his whooshing and started making weird noises.

'Ya hah hey a ya ha heya, heya heya yata heya.'

He repeated this a few times, finishing each passage with a dramatic, 'Yaheya!' It sounded like some sort of Native American incantation. Had I slipped through a wormhole and onto the set of *F Troop*? Was Alan the lost member of the Hekawi tribe? Then, suddenly, he ceased chanting and went back to whooshing.

It would have all seemed a little odd, I imagine, to anyone passing – you could easily see in from the scuzzy street outside – but I was so relaxed I didn't care. I drifted off into a sort of reverie while Alan continued to work me over in his funny little way. Then when I was, I think, on the verge of falling asleep he turned the music off and I opened my eyes. He passed his hands over me a couple more times and said: 'You're cooked.'

'Right,' I said, rubbing my face.

'How do you feel?'

'Um, I feel fine, I think,' I said. 'Hard to say, really. But I think I feel a bit better.' I felt I should say that because he seemed like a nice guy. I didn't want to hurt his feelings by telling him I would probably feel the same effect after an hour at home on the couch.

'You should feel better,' he said. 'We've done quite a bit of clearing there. I think you'll notice a big difference.'

'Yes, sure, thanks,' I said, putting my shoes and socks back on. I forked over my $80, shook him by the hand and went out to my car. As I was getting in, I saw a well-known TV personality and actress who'd starred in any number of awful soaps pulling up behind me. She looked around furtively then got out and went into Alan's with a scarf pulled over her head. I'd found my own celebrity healer! I made a mental note to tell Sandra about this — it would make a great scoop for *TV Week*.

Now I wasn't sure what Alan had done to me or for me, but I did actually feel better. Part of me suspected he was a charlatan, and that part also suspected he rented this nondescript house on a short-term lease and would probably move from place to place to keep one step ahead of *A Current Affair*. But if he was a fake, how could you prove it? He at least seemed a genuine fake because he engendered a sense of calm in his client. I really did feel energised, and I suspended my disbelief in this case.

I went straight to pick Sandra up from work.

'So tell me, what exactly did this guy do to you?' she asked.

'Hard to say really,' I said. 'It was all very subtle.'

'How much did this subtlety cost?'

'Eighty bucks.'

'You could have had a damn good Shiatsu massage for that.'

'Yes, but I do feel better,' I promised.

Secretly, I went back the following week and had another session with Alan, who did much the same thing... lots of whooshing and plenty of chanting and deep breathing, which apparently helps distribute chi (they all talk about chi). Several sessions later the treatment was still the same. As I lay there, I wondered what he did with his money because his digs were pretty rudimentary and he wasn't exactly a fashion plate. He always wore the same jeans and a plain, slightly grubby white T-shirt. There were no outward signs of prosperity, yet there was always someone hot on my heels after each session and often someone leaving as I arrived. He must have been making hundreds of dollars a day.

After five sessions he declared me cured – which was just as well, because Sandra found out I'd been going back to him and was on at me about the expense.

'Everything's flowing freely now,' he said, pleased with himself. 'I don't think you'll have any more problems.' It was a big call but he seemed sure. And, strangely, the midnight waking and the malarial sweats had subsided during this treatment. Sandra was convinced this was just nature taking its course and that whatever bug I'd got from the dreaded plate of seafood noodles I'd eaten that fateful night on Tioman had been expunged from my system in the normal course of events.

Anyway, I was happy to be sleeping nights again, whether it was Alan's whooshing that had cured me or otherwise.

About a year later I was driving over St Kilda way and I decided to go down his street again, just for curiosity's sake. I pulled up in front of the place and was surprised to see it all boarded up. Intrigued, I rang his number when I got home and it seemed to be disconnected. I had no idea what that meant but it seemed a bit weird.

'Don't you think it's spooky?' I asked Sandra.

'Nothing spooky about that,' she said. 'He's probably living in the Cayman Islands now.'

'Good on him,' I said. 'He cured me.'

'Yeah, right,' Sandra said.

The Future, Now

Anxiety neurosis doesn't like a cure. It's a condition that abhors its host feeling well. So, despite being apparently cured in Melbourne, I was slowly building up a head of steam, angst-wise, about my health again. We'd moved back to Brisbane, and I'd started getting headaches and my tummy was playing up a bit. We had settled back into life in the subtropical Queensland capital and things were going well professionally: I had a good job at *Brisbane News*, a lifestyle magazine (did this mean Brisbane actually had a lifestyle? some southern friends asked). But it's when things are going well – despite the minor flaws of the flesh – that one worries most, because the obvious corollary of everything running smoothly is that there must be some bumps ahead.

Consequently, I was worried about the future. But as a friend says – yesterday's history, tomorrow's a mystery, and there's not much you can do about that, is there? Or . . . is there? Whenever I've had questions about the future, I like to get answers. That's what clairvoyants are for, after all, and in between all my other dabblings I have been known to explore the future with a little help from the odd fortune teller. And as my anxiety began to build again – related to nothing in particular, other than the fact that I was alive, and therefore anxious – I sought solace in a seer. Which brought me to an appointment with the latest in a long line of soothsayers.

The door of room 26 opened to reveal a short, dishevelled, bearded bloke wearing drawstring trousers and a soiled T-shirt. I had been buzzed up from the foyer for my consultation with a visiting clairvoyant, but this didn't look like him. At a second glance I was almost sure I had, instead, disturbed the singer Brian Cadd. The beard fitted. Then, from within the beard, came a greeting: 'You must be Phil.'

I offered my hand, asking tentatively, 'Darren?' Not the most auspicious name for a clairvoyant, I felt. I would have preferred something a bit more exotic . . . say, Algernon or Hercule. But half of me was still hoping this was Brian Cadd – or anyone but my clairvoyant.

I love clairvoyants. If there is such a thing as a 'future junkie', I suppose I was one. It was something about the excitement of the unknown and the possibility of wonderful things in store that made the future so addictive.

I had come at the suggestion of a friend with a mutual interest in soothsaying – that is, someone similarly insecure and always on the hunt for good news about the future. My friend had rung me from Sydney to spruik her latest find, the 'incredible' Darren, a seer who travelled the eastern seaboard divining people's futures – for a price. She had found him helpful, she said, so I thought I'd give him a whirl since he was in Brisbane for a few days. The nondescript motel he was holed up at was the sort of joint you'd expect travelling salespeople or faded rock stars on leagues club tours to frequent. But I tried hard to keep an open mind, even though the combination of his name, his looks and his travelling 'office' spelt doom from the start. Still, I was here for his genius, not the atmosphere, I told myself – again.

I had a mid-morning appointment for my reading and had slipped out of the office after writing 'Gone to a doctor's appointment' on the whiteboard. I usually had a weekly doctor's appointment, anyway, so it's not as if anyone would have been surprised.

Darren and Brian Cadd must surely have been separated at birth, I thought as I sat opposite him at a small, wonky table, trying not to focus on the food remnants stuck in his beard.

As we sat, he closed his eyes and started talking at a rapid pace. 'You're sensitive, you're very sensitive, I can feel that,' he murmured, turning his head from side to side as he spoke. 'Much too sensitive for your own good. Much too sensitive... But you are practical, too, and very creative. Too creative for the work you're doing, oh yes, definitely. You write, don't you? I can see that but it's not for you. No, no. You should be scriptwriting, yes, that's it... scriptwriting for films. Los Angeles. Hollywood. That's where you need to be. Right where it's happening. America, that's where it will happen for you, I can see that. America. I can see that very clearly.'

He paused for a millisecond but then he was off again, before I could get him to expand on the possibility of fame, women and lots of American dollars. 'You have to watch your health,' he chanted. 'Watch your health indeed. You must drink more water. Less coffee, more water, and when you take those tablets you take... swallow them with more water. Much more water. Better for your kidneys. Much better. Will also keep those headaches at bay.'

This was very boring, but accurate.

'The headaches come because you're not doing what the universe wants you to do. Nowhere near enough creativity happening. That's a problem. That's a big problem. Have to get in tune with the universe, follow your fate.' There was a silence, and then he opened his eyes. 'Did I say something?' he asked, looking a bit dazed. 'Spontaneous. Totally spontaneous. Never remember a word of it afterwards. It comes from the source, unbidden, flowing.'

'Really?' I tried to sound impressed but I already had my doubts. In fact I had no desire at all to go to America, for a start, so his prediction could be tricky. Couldn't I just win Lotto and move to Noosa?

'Shuffle the cards and cut them, please,' he said, so I picked up the Tarot deck between us and did so. I cut the cards, chose six, and he laid them out on the table. Then he was off again, muttering through his beard, drifting into an apparent half-trance while I tried to latch on to anything that sounded even vaguely attractive. I'd had good Tarot readings before and was hoping for something special this time.

My ears pricked up finally when he suggested I would be coming into some money. The universe really did want to provide for me without the necessity of having to work, I was sure of that. Never mind that a string of clairvoyants had already predicted windfalls with no result.

But Darren just didn't give off much of a psychic vibe. He still looked like an old rocker down on his luck, and when he opened his mouth I was sure he was going to sing 'A Little Ray of Sunshine'. Instead I got some malarky about not responding to offers of assistance from a tall man with a mole on his right cheek.

'Jesus, that's pretty specific,' I said when he'd tuned back in.

'Sometimes things are general, cloudy, but other times clear as day. Something comes in from the ether,' he explained, adding: 'It's all a mystery, all a mystery.'

Wrapped in a riddle and tossed lightly with a green salad and rip-off sauce. I mean, I like a good reading as much as the next desperado, but this guy hadn't seemed kosher from the moment he started in on me.

With that, the session seemed to be over, and before I knew it Darren was ushering me out the door after separating me from a crisp new $100 bill. Then I was crossing the foyer, where a nervous young woman sat flicking through a copy of *Woman's Day*.

'He's ready for you now,' the receptionist said. The girl

got up and was buzzed through to the lift. P T Barnum was right, I thought, there is one born every minute.

I went back to work disgruntled and sat at my desk annoyed that I'd spent good money for no real result. I phoned my wife, Sandra, to report in.

'Any good news?' she asked.

'Not unless you want to pack everything now and move to Los Angeles, where fame and fortune await,' I scoffed.

'No way,' she said. 'What a load of old codswallop. What else did he say?'

'That I was going on a long sea voyage and would meet a tall dark stranger.'

'Really?'

'No, not really.'

I found it hard to explain why I kept going back for more. I told myself it was because I was – despite evidence to the contrary – an optimist, certain something incredible was just around the corner. Of course, being a nervous kind of chap, I knew I'd cope better if I just knew when it'd be coming. I mean, who wouldn't want to be prepared?

Growing up in Hong Kong had probably softened me up for accepting the idea of dabbling. The Cantonese are a superstitious lot and regularly consult astrologers and fortune tellers. I remember watching these seers plying their trade on the streets of Kowloon. Perhaps the strangest practitioner was one I encountered at Shau Kei Wan on Hong Kong Island in the 1980s. I was visiting my aunt and uncle. My uncle, Cyril, was in charge of the engineering works of a section of the MTR rail system, which was being built at the time. He was working on the Shau Kei Wan section a few kilometres east of the famous Star Ferry, in an area that was still very traditional and a world away from the high-rise towers of Central. In a street near my uncle's site office, a blind fortune teller plied his trade, reading people's futures from the grooves in tortoise shells. I had heard of tea-leaf reading and people who divined things from the palms of hands or bumps on the head, but this was a newie to me.

'Why don't you have a go?' prompted my uncle as we sauntered past one lunchtime on a mission to find the perfect bowl of noodles.

'No way,' I said. 'I don't like the look of that tortoise.' Besides, the fellow's stall — which consisted of a stool and a basket of live tortoises — was situated right next to a coffin shop. The open caskets were propped outside the door, right on the street. I guess it pays to advertise. I wasn't sure how much passing trade they got, but I suspected the blind bloke and the coffin salesman might be in cahoots, so I passed on by.

I did have my fortune told in Singapore a few years later, when a cab driver decided to do an unsolicited reading during a ride across town.

'You are writer,' he said, as a matter of fact. It was probably the whiff of insolvency that tipped him.

'Well, I'm a journalist,' I said, feeling uncomfortable about any literary pretensions.

'No, you are writer too,' he said. I was a published poet as well, so he wasn't exactly wrong. My ears pricked up.

'Success may come to you later in life,' he said. 'That is how I see it.' This seer, stuck behind the wheel in the freezing cabin of his taxi, made a few other interesting predictions and insights en route to Chinatown.

Back home, I began to consult the occasional clairvoyant, usually a woman. Disappointingly, like Darren, they never seemed very exotic creatures. With names like Shirley or Raelene, they would invariably call you 'Darl' and say 'youse' a lot. I became adept at hunting them down in those funny little shops that sell crystals and incense down the end of run-down arcades or at market stalls (I've seen some of them even using crystal balls!) or working from home in the desiccated outer suburbs. When we were living in Melbourne, I used to intermittently visit a woman called Anne who lived in a brick-veneer suburban wilderness, a long haul from our digs in the trendy inner city.

Anne was a quiet, immaculately-groomed woman with an impressive ability to get to the heart of the matter, although she too had the 'youse' disease. I always left satisfied with her insights and what she picked up on, never begrudging her the fee. I put it down to 'personal growth' and didn't stint on the budget. Sometimes I'd play the tapes of our sessions back a few years later only to find that another of her predictions had come true. She had pinpointed the month of our shift back to Brisbane, actually – something I'd forgotten in the hectic whirl of the move. But when I played back her tape after digging it out of a box of stuff a while later, it was all there, along with all sorts of other little nuances of detail that seemed to fit. If you'd passed

Anne at the supermarket, though, she'd look like any suburban housewife filling her trolley rather than someone who had a direct line to the other side.

I guess you have to believe that there is another dimension before you go calling on a clairvoyant. And you have to believe that some people can plug into it and download information from that vast continuum, eternity, where all time exists in one time, where everything that is and will be is known. No matter what they look like.

People have believed this sort of stuff for aeons, and history is full of examples of decisive action taken after consulting soothsayers. Alexander the Great's rise was predicted, and in ancient Greece the Delphic Oracle was often consulted by the high and mighty. The Romans were keen on it, too, and tried to divine the future from the flights of birds or the entrails of beasts. So I felt I was following in a fine tradition – but Sandra tended to disagree, especially when I overspent on my addiction or got caught in a palm-reader's clutches when I'd been sent to get something urgently at the supermarket.

After moving back to Brissie, I found it hard to replace Anne. Getting hold of a really reliable clairvoyant wasn't easy – until I finally happened upon Margaret Bowman. I had a recommendation to consult her at a time when I was particularly desperate. Sandra and I were heading overseas on a major European jaunt and I needed confirmation from a reliable source, besides the airline, that the plane would actually reach its destination – London's Heathrow – without falling out of the sky. I was serious about this.

So I rang Margaret to make an appointment to get assurances about the trip. She lived just a few kilometres from my office.

'Would you like me to come over for the reading?' I asked.

'No, we can just do it on the phone,' she replied.

Now don't think for a moment that Margaret is like those dial-up services that people use for sex chats or astrological readings. She assured me that by the timbre of my voice, visualisation and various communications — she wasn't specific about with whom she'd be communicating — she could read as accurately as if I was sitting in front of her. This required a certain suspension of disbelief, but I was quite prepared to do that to get the result I was after.

For this first consultation, I had very specific questions. 'Basically, the first thing I want to ask is — will I survive the flight?'

'Can you give me the flight details?' she asked. I referred to the itinerary and gave her the flight numbers, departure and arrival times.

'Just a minute, I'll ask them,' she said. I heard her mumbling in the background for a little while in a voice that was at once both insistent and deferential. Then I recalled that I had been warned about this, that she talked to dead people: those who dwell with us, unseen. I thought it was a joke at first, but it was no joke. After that, Margaret gave some quite specific details about the flight — weather and so on — which proved to be pretty accurate, although I'm sure any sceptic would rationalise each and every one of them.

But one of her predictions was so spot-on, it was uncanny: she predicted that before landing, the captain would come out of the cockpit and greet us, and that he would be drinking a mug of tea.

That didn't actually happen until we had crossed the English coast. We were upstairs in Business Class and out popped this tall, distinguished-looking man, mug of tea in his mitt — just as Margaret had suggested.

'Jolly nice morning,' he said, sounding like a Battle of Britain squadron leader. It was a small but impressive detail.

When we landed at Heathrow I turned to Sandra and said: 'Margaret was right about something else too.'

'What do you mean?' she said.

'We did survive the flight!'

'*Everyone* survived the flight,' said Sandra with a glare. 'Ninety-nine percent of the time they do.'

When we got back, I started phoning Margaret whenever we flew. As soon as a flight was booked and I had an itinerary, I would dial her up to check my survivability rating. The outcome was always positive, although occasionally there'd be a bit of niggling information, something like, 'You'll experience turbulence fifteen minutes out of Sydney', which we would; or, 'When you arrive in Townsville there will be a light drizzle', and there was, even though it hardly ever rains in Townsville. Not the sort of thing that would convince a sceptic, but I was sold.

Naturally, Margaret charges for her readings, and a few days afterwards a fee would pop up on my credit card bill.

Sandra complained that I was spending too much on this indulgence, but I found Margaret's assurances comforting and the advice that came with the readings helpful — if a bit addictive.

I was impressed, too, with the fact that she had some rather famous people on her books and that she had an international profile. She'd pop off to places like Dubai and Hong Kong occasionally, set herself up in some hotel, and see a string of rich expats who probably had nothing better to do than worry about their money.

Margaret had some impressive successes, including an episode in which she had pointed some historians in the direction of the last campsite of some colonial explorers who disappeared in the Northern Territory sometime in the nineteenth century. Margaret located the site, and bones were eventually found there, confirming that the explorers had come to a bitter end in the middle of nowhere.

I was hooked, and found myself ringing Margaret more often than I should. I'd be in the office trying to talk in hushed tones so nobody knew what I was up to. If I was feeling a bit squiffy, I'd ring, and she would seem to be able to pinpoint the problem exactly. If it was to do with office politics, she seemed to be able to read the situation with amazing clarity. How did she do that down the phone? Not sure about that, but it was working for me and I'm glad it was.

When I had a few more rumbles than usual in the tummy one day, I decided to ask Margaret about it.

'I think you should go and see a doctor,' she said.

'You think it's something serious?' I gasped.

'Just a minute.' I heard her asking for guidance. Who, on the other side, could really give a stuff about my bowels?

'No, we don't think it's serious but we must check anyway,' she came back.

This sent me into a bit of a tailspin, so I tore off to see my local GP with a deeply furrowed brow. When he asked what prompted my visit, I was going to tell him about my clairvoyant, but thought better of that and just said I'd had some ominous rumblings in the nether regions and I was concerned.

He referred me on to a gastroenterologist, a dapper man whose rooms were adorned with antiquarian etchings. He was obviously trying to create an atmosphere in his chambers that could distract him from the grim reality of his work: that is, sticking his hand up people's bums all day. When he led me into the small cubicle – a very nice, wood-panelled cubicle – attached to his office, I was afraid, very afraid. And there was a moment when, in the degrading minutes that followed, I did want to ask: 'Does this mean we're engaged?'

The upside of the experience was that I felt very relieved when it was all over. He found nothing obviously wrong but decided to send me off for a more thorough investigation.

'Normally I wouldn't take this any further, but I think you need a little more convincing than some of my patients,' he said, smiling.

After a week spent living on my nerve ends, I presented myself at a hospital in Brisbane's north for a virtual colonoscopy, during which I was basically filled with air and x-rayed. For this process you have to wear one of those back-to-front gowns, which you have to walk around in beforehand looking like a real goose (but at least I knew how they worked, thanks to Gunther and his colonic irrigation clinic!). My humiliation was complete when a nurse pumped me up like a bicycle tyre and shoved me through the x-ray machine.

'When will I get the results?' I asked when I was dressed again.

'Your doctor should have them in a few days,' I was told.

Which was fine. Or was it? I had felt confident about the test and Margaret had said she felt it would be okay, but had she been as emphatic as usual? I thought not. So I rang her afterwards to find out and got her answering machine. Then I rang her mobile and got no response. Had she gone overseas again? I sweated it out for a few days waiting for the results. I rang the doctor's rooms a couple of times to see if the results were back, but couldn't get a straight answer out of the receptionist. Specialists' receptionists won't tell you anything, and when you ask to speak to the doctor you're met with incredulity.

'The doctor is far too busy,' I was told. 'He's with patients all day.'

'But I'm a patient too, and he did say to ring about the results,' I pleaded.

'Yes, but we can't just put through everyone who rings,' she chided.

I could just see him with his hand up someone as we

spoke. Undeterred, I rang back several more times until finally the receptionist weakened and admitted that, 'The doctor has the results and will call you about them later.' He had the results? He'd call me later? Why wouldn't he speak with me now? Was it such bad news that he needed the whole day to steel himself for it? Did he want to be sitting quietly in his empty rooms at the end of the day to give me the awful prognosis?

I re-dialled Margaret immediately. I wanted the future and I wanted it now! I couldn't wait until the afternoon. Even though my desk is underneath an airconditioning vent and I spend much of my time in the office fighting off hypothermia, I felt hot and clammy. The good news was that Margaret's phone wasn't ringing out any more. It went to voice mail, which meant, I was sure, that she was in the country and available. I tried the mobile again too, but got voice mail there too. I left a message. 'I need to speak with you urgently about a matter of the utmost importance,' I said, trying to keep my voice down so my colleagues couldn't hear. I tried to work, but found myself staring vacantly at the computer. I tried the doctor again but the receptionist fobbed me off, quite angrily this time.

'I told you he'll call you after he's seen his last patient,' she said.

'When will that be?' I insisted.

'Around 5 p.m.'

I felt it could be all over by then. I was now terrified. What would he say? 'Mr Brown, don't make any plans for Christmas'? I was too young to die, or at least too unprepared.

I had a lot more television to watch before I was ready to join Margaret's friends over yonder. I rang her again and left what I hoped sounded like a desperate message for her to call me urgently on a matter pertaining to my future. Mind you, that was standard fare for her, so I rang again and said I couldn't make it through the next few hours without some sort of certitude regarding a matter we had discussed in the not-too-distant past. No reply. I sat at the desk, the words blurring on the screen in front of me. I rang Sandra, who said what any normal wife would say: 'Don't be so bloody silly, the doctor's just busy. I'm sure it will be okay.' Which is fine – but then, she's no clairvoyant.

The minutes passed like glaciers that afternoon, and several more calls to Margaret were unsuccessful. By 4.30 p.m. I was mentally composing a deathbed speech. Twenty minutes later the phone on my desk rang and I picked it up with a snatching motion.

'Hello, Mr Brown?' a voice said.

'Yes,' I whimpered.

'Dr Simpson here.' Oh, God, him. Just then my mobile started ringing.

'You have some news for me?' I croaked. Just then I looked down and saw that the number flashing on the mobile was Margaret's.

'Doctor, can you excuse me for one moment while I take this other call?' He did so reluctantly.

'Hello, Margaret. I've got the doctor on the other line with my results.'

'The results are all clear,' she said. 'I've just got an answer on that myself.' Her source was a little less empirical than the doctor's, but I felt a wave of relief sweep over me.

'You're 100 percent certain of that?' I asked.

'They never lie,' she said. I guess you're not allowed to over there, up there or wherever it is.

I picked up the handset of my landline again. 'Hello, doctor?'

'Mr Brown, yes, well I just rang to say I have your test results here and everything seems fine.'

'Yes, yes, doctor, thanks very much for getting back to me.' I felt like telling him that a second or two earlier I'd had confirmation of all this from the spirit world, but that wasn't something he needed to know.

'Thanks for that, that's great news,' I said.

'Hopefully that will put your mind at rest,' he said. 'For a while at least.'

'Yes, thank you, goodbye, doctor.'

I went back to Margaret. 'So everything's looking good, they reckon?'

'Yes, although they do say you need to stop worrying so much.'

I felt the sort of temporary elation that usually follows a life-threatening situation – one that you survive.

Recently, when Margaret was away on an overseas trip, I weakened and consulted another psychic, a woman called Suzie. (I did mention that I was addicted, didn't I?) She worked from a small cluttered room behind a New Age shop in an area that looked like it might have produced its fair share of serial killers. I felt like I was cheating on

Margaret by seeing her, but I was feeling a bit wonky and someone had suggested Suzie. Besides, I was desperate, so I'm sure if I ever mention it to Margaret (which I won't), she'll understand.

Before the reading, she insisted on giving me a full body scan by running her hands down the front of my body to check my aura (I hoped she knew where it began and ended). Having done this and cleared a few 'chakras' en route, she communed with the world beyond via various entities. She had trouble communicating with my dead rellies — mainly, she said, because she felt that most of them, being Catholic, didn't want any part of such spiritual shenanigans. Except a late aunty who apparently popped by just to say hello. There were some other less specific spirits floating around during the session, and as each one appeared Suzie would welcome them, and after their words of wisdom had been shared she'd tell them, gently, to push off back to whatever level of the after-life they had attained.

'We thank youse for coming by,' Suzie intoned, 'but we ask youse to leave us now, spirits, and be on your way.'

I felt the urge to wave them off too, and as she closed her eyes and thanked the universe for being there, I wondered which of us was the bigger loony.

It was at this point that it dawned on me how utterly mad she was. Or was it just me? I mean, how does a supposedly intelligent, verging-on-middle-aged man end up in the back room of a dowdy New Age shop having his aura read by a spirit-channelling suburban mum? Life, it gets weird sometimes.

As I was wondering about this, she began making flicking gestures around me.

'Just clearing ya energy field,' she said.

'Are they gone?' I asked when she sat down again.

'Yep, all gone and happy as Larry,' she said, clicking off the small, rickety tape recorder on which she'd been recording the session.

'Here you go, you'll probably have forgotten a lot of this by the time you get home but ya can play it back later,' she said.

I forked over the $80 fee and left her to it. She had another customer waiting outside, a woman who almost knocked me over going in as I came out. Talk about desperate.

I, meanwhile, went to the small, tatty bakery next door and got an apple slice to fortify myself for the drive back to the inner city. I was keen to get home because I was supposed to be there writing a book review I'd taken the day off to complete. I hadn't told Sandra I was going for a reading because I knew she'd be annoyed that I was spending more money on divining my future.

Of course, everything Suzie said may have been absolute rubbish, I thought as I drove home. The more I thought about this, the crazier the whole thing seemed. How could someone I've never seen before in my entire life have any idea about my future? Wasn't a man master of his own destiny? Wasn't life to be lived in the here and now? Wasn't the future a mystery to be lived rather than a problem to be solved? Wasn't it time I just got on with it and stopped dilly-dallying around? I remembered what Dr Reeve had said to me once — this wasn't a dress rehearsal.

So when I got home I chucked the cassette into the bin. It was liberating. I felt empowered! I'm in charge of me, I thought. And today is the beginning of the rest of my life. No more clairvoyants, no more remedies, no more gurus – just me and the future of endless possibilities.

I made a mental note to ring Margaret as soon as she returned to find out what they might be.

Acknowledgements

Huge thanks to my publisher, Madonna Duffy, for her guidance and friendship. To senior editor, Anna Crago, who was so great to work with, suitably firm and very clear about how things should be, which helped a lot. To Greg Bain and the rest of the team – authors talk about the UQP family, and now I know what they mean. To Sean Doyle for his meticulous editing, sense of humour and willingness to do a bit of workshopping along the way with a confused author. To Ben Robertson and Liz Johnston for reading early stories and giving honest feedback. To Alison Walsh who cast her sub-editor's eye over the first draft. To Ross Fitzgerald, Manfred Jurgensen and Margaret Bowman for moral support. Thanks also to Bruce Dawe and Les Murray for agreeing to be included. And to Sandy Cull for a bright, brilliant cover.

Particular thanks to my wife, Sandra McLean, for reading the stories as they were written, for being honest about the work in progress, and for putting up with evening absences.

Also to my mum, Janet McLaren Brown, for being there for me during some wacky times.

They say if you can remember the Sixties, you weren't really there, and perhaps the same can be said, to a degree at least, about some parts of the Seventies and Eighties. The memory may be fuzzy at times but I'm pretty sure it all really happened. However, some of the characters and events have been changed for dramatic effect.